# HEALTHY GLUTEN-FREE VEGAN LIFESTYLE

## Over 100 Delicious & Healthy Dairy-Free Recipes (Breakfast, Lunch, Dinner, Dessert & Snacks) For Beginners

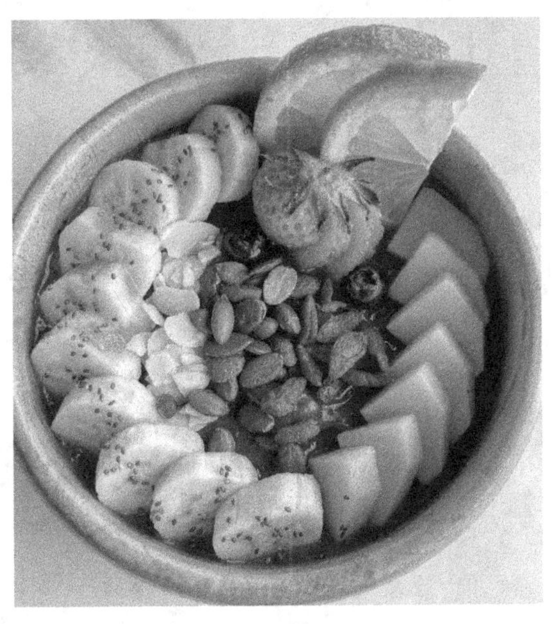

## Grace Ashley

# TABLE OF CONTENT

# INTRODUCTION

In recent years, the gluten-free vegan lifestyle has gained significant attention as individuals seek to improve their health, address dietary sensitivities, and embrace ethical eating practices. This lifestyle choice combines the principles of a gluten-free diet, which excludes gluten-containing grains like wheat, barley, and rye, with the tenets of veganism, which eschews all animal products.

## Understanding Gluten and the Gluten-Free Diet

Gluten is a protein found in Berley, Wheat, rye, and their derivatives. For individuals with celiac disease, an autoimmune disorder affecting about 1% of the population, consuming gluten triggers an immune response that damages the small intestine. Additionally, some individuals may have non-celiac gluten sensitivity, experiencing gastrointestinal discomfort and other symptoms after gluten consumption without the autoimmune component.

The gluten-free diet involves eliminating all sources of gluten from one's meals and snacks. This requires careful scrutiny of ingredient labels, as gluten can hide in unexpected places such as sauces, seasonings, and processed foods.

# Medical Conditions and Gluten

Gluten is a protein found in wheat, barley, rye, and sometimes oats. For most people, consuming gluten poses no significant health risks. However, for individuals with certain medical conditions, gluten can trigger adverse reactions, leading to a range of symptoms and complications. Two primary medical conditions associated with gluten are celiac disease and non-celiac gluten sensitivity (NCGS). Additionally, wheat allergy is another condition related to gluten ingestion, although it differs from celiac disease and NCGS in its underlying mechanisms and clinical manifestations.

Celiac Disease:

Celiac disease is an autoimmune disorder characterized by an abnormal immune response to gluten ingestion, resulting in inflammation and damage to the lining of the small intestine. This damage impairs nutrient absorption and can lead to various gastrointestinal symptoms, such as diarrhea, abdominal pain, bloating, and malnutrition. However, celiac disease can also manifest with non-gastrointestinal symptoms, including fatigue, joint pain, skin rash (dermatitis herpetiformis), and neurological issues.
Long-term complications of untreated celiac disease can be severe and include osteoporosis, infertility, neurological disorders, and an increased risk of certain cancers. The only effective treatment for celiac disease is strict adherence to a gluten-free diet, which involves avoiding all sources of gluten-containing grains.

Non-Celiac Gluten Sensitivity (NCGS):

NCGS is a condition characterized by adverse reactions to gluten ingestion in individuals who do not have celiac disease or wheat allergy. The exact mechanisms underlying NCGS are not fully understood, but it is believed to involve a combination of immune, genetic, and environmental factors. Symptoms of NCGS are similar to those of celiac disease and may include gastrointestinal discomfort, bloating, diarrhea, fatigue, headaches, and joint pain.

Unlike celiac disease, NCGS does not cause damage to the small intestine, and there are currently no specific diagnostic tests for the condition. Diagnosis is typically made through the exclusion of celiac disease and wheat allergy followed by a trial of a gluten-free diet to assess symptom improvement. Management of NCGS involves avoiding gluten-containing foods, although the long-term implications and prognosis of the condition remain areas of ongoing research.

Wheat Allergy:

Wheat allergy is an immune-mediated reaction to proteins found in wheat, including but not limited to gluten. Unlike celiac disease and NCGS, which involve abnormal immune responses, wheat allergy is characterized by the production of IgE antibodies against wheat proteins, leading to allergic symptoms upon exposure.

Symptoms of wheat allergy can vary widely and may include skin reactions (such as hives or eczema), respiratory symptoms (such as wheezing or nasal congestion), gastrointestinal symptoms (such as nausea or vomiting), and, in severe cases, anaphylaxis. Diagnosis is typically based on a combination of medical history, physical examination, and allergy testing (such as skin prick tests or blood tests). Management involves strict avoidance of wheat and wheat-derived products, with prompt treatment of allergic reactions if they occur.

In conclusion, while gluten-related medical conditions vary in their underlying mechanisms and clinical presentations, they all necessitate strict avoidance of gluten-containing foods to prevent symptoms and complications. For individuals diagnosed with celiac disease, NCGS, or wheat allergy, adopting a gluten-free diet is crucial for managing their condition and maintaining optimal health and well-being. Additionally, ongoing research into the pathogenesis and treatment of these conditions is essential for improving diagnostic accuracy, developing targeted therapies, and enhancing the quality of life for affected individuals.

## Why Go Gluten-Free?

There are several reasons why individuals may choose to adopt a gluten-free lifestyle:

Health Benefits: For those with celiac disease or NCGS, eliminating gluten is essential for managing symptoms and preventing long-term complications.

Improved Digestion: Some people find that reducing or eliminating gluten from their diet alleviates digestive discomfort such as bloating, gas, and irregular bowel movements.

Weight Management: Going gluten-free may lead to weight loss for some individuals, particularly if they replace gluten-containing processed foods with whole, nutrient-dense alternatives.

Enhanced Energy Levels: Eliminating gluten may help some people experience increased energy levels and improved overall well-being.

## Foods to Consume and Meal Planning

Following a gluten-free vegan diet requires careful planning to ensure adequate nutrition and variety. Here are some gluten-free vegan-friendly foods to include:

- Fruits and vegetables
- Legumes (beans, lentils, chickpeas)
- Nuts and seeds
- Gluten-free whole grains (quinoa, rice, millet, amaranth)
- Gluten-free flours (Coconut flour, Chickpea flour, Almond flour)
- Plant-based protein sources (tofu, tempeh, seitan)

A well-balanced gluten-free vegan meal plan might include:

- Breakfast: Quinoa porridge with almond milk, topped with fresh berries and nuts
- Lunch: Lentil and vegetable soup with a side salad dressed with olive oil and lemon juice
- Dinner: Brown rice served with Stir-fried vegetables and Tofu
- Snacks: Raw vegetables with hummus, fruit with nut butter, or gluten-free crackers with avocado

## Foods to Avoid

When following a gluten-free vegan lifestyle, it's important to steer clear of foods containing gluten as well as animal-derived products. Foods to avoid include:

- Wheat, barley, rye, and their derivatives (bread, pasta, cereal, baked goods)
- Processed foods with hidden gluten (sauces, dressings, marinades)
- Animal products (meat, dairy, eggs, honey)
- Cross-contaminated foods (products processed in facilities that also handle gluten-containing ingredients)

---

By adopting a gluten-free vegan lifestyle, individuals can enjoy a diverse and flavorful array of plant-based foods while supporting their health and ethical values. With careful planning and creativity in the kitchen, navigating this dietary approach can be both fulfilling and rewarding.

Creating gluten-free vegan recipes requires a thoughtful approach to ensure both delicious flavor and nutritional balance. Here are some key characteristics of such recipes, along with information on essential ingredients and cooking techniques:

1. Emphasis on Whole Foods: Gluten-free vegan recipes often focus on whole, minimally processed ingredients such as fruits, vegetables, legumes, nuts, seeds, and gluten-free grains. These nutrient-dense foods form the foundation of a balanced diet and provide essential vitamins, minerals, fiber, and antioxidants.

2. Alternative Flours and Binders: In place of wheat flour, gluten-free recipes utilize a variety of alternative flours such as almond flour, coconut flour, rice flour, chickpea flour, and tapioca flour. These flours impart unique flavors and textures to dishes while providing gluten-free options for baking, thickening sauces, and coating ingredients. Additionally, vegan binders such as ground flaxseeds, chia seeds, psyllium husk, and arrowroot powder are often used to replace eggs in recipes, helping to bind ingredients together and achieve desired textures.

3. Plant-Based Protein Sources: To ensure adequate protein intake, gluten-free vegan recipes incorporate a variety of plant-based protein sources such as tofu, tempeh, seitan, lentils, beans, and quinoa. These ingredients not only provide essential amino acids but also contribute to the overall flavor, texture, and satiety of dishes.

4. Creative Flavor Profiles: Gluten-free vegan cooking encourages creativity in flavor profiles, drawing inspiration from global cuisines and a diverse array of herbs, spices, condiments, and sauces. Ingredients such as nutritional yeast, tamari, miso paste, tahini, coconut aminos, and curry pastes add depth and complexity to dishes, enhancing their appeal and satisfying the palate.

5. Focus on Texture and Mouthfeel: Texture plays a crucial role in gluten-free vegan cooking, as many gluten-free flours and ingredients behave differently from traditional wheat-based counterparts. Recipes often incorporate techniques such as soaking, sprouting, blending, and fermenting to achieve desired textures and improve digestibility. Additionally, ingredients such as aquafaba (the liquid from canned chickpeas), agar-agar, and tapioca starch are used to create elasticity, moisture, and structure in baked goods and other dishes.

6. Allergen Awareness: Gluten-free vegan recipes prioritize allergen awareness and accommodate individuals with dietary restrictions or sensitivities. Careful attention is paid to cross-contamination risks, and alternative ingredients are used to replace common allergens such as wheat, soy, dairy, and nuts. Recipes may include allergen-free substitutions and variations to cater to diverse dietary needs and preferences.

7. Versatility and Adaptability: Gluten-free vegan recipes are versatile and adaptable, allowing for customization based on ingredient availability, seasonality, and personal taste preferences. Cooks are encouraged to experiment with substitutions, variations, and creative

twists to make dishes their own while staying true to the principles of gluten-free and vegan cooking.

## Essential Ingredients:

- Alternative flours (almond flour, coconut flour, rice flour, etc.)
- Plant-based protein sources (tofu, tempeh, lentils, beans, quinoa, etc.)
- Gluten-free grains (quinoa, rice, millet, amaranth, etc.)
- Vegan binders (ground flaxseeds, chia seeds, psyllium husk, arrowroot powder, etc.)
- Nutritional yeast
- Tamari or gluten-free soy sauce
- Miso paste
- Tahini
- Coconut aminos
- Curry pastes
- Aquafaba (chickpea brine)
- Agar-agar
- Tapioca starch

## Cooking Techniques:

- Baking: Using alternative flours and binders to create gluten-free baked goods such as bread, cakes, cookies, and muffins.
- Sauteing and Stir-Frying: Cooking vegetables, tofu, tempeh, and other ingredients in a skillet or wok with oil, herbs, spices, and sauces.
- Steaming: Cooking grains, vegetables, and dumplings by exposing them to steam in a covered pot or steamer basket.

- Boiling and Simmering: Preparing soups, stews, grains, and legumes in liquid over low to medium heat until tender and flavorful.
- Blending and Pureeing: Creating smoothies, sauces, dips, and creamy textures using a blender or food processor.
- Fermenting: Cultivating beneficial bacteria and enzymes in foods such as tempeh, miso, sauerkraut, and kimchi to enhance flavor and digestibility.

By incorporating these characteristics, essential ingredients, and cooking techniques into gluten-free vegan recipes, cooks can create delicious, nutritious, and satisfying meals that cater to a diverse range of tastes and dietary needs.

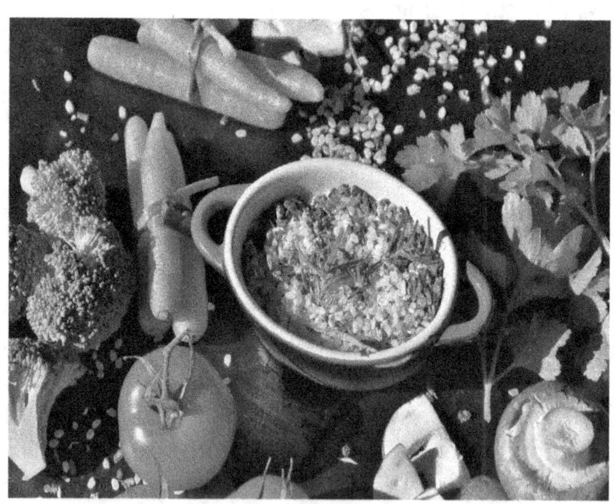

# RECIPES



BREAKFAST

1. Quinoa Breakfast Bowl

Ingredients:

- 1/2 cup cooked quinoa
- 1/2 cup mixed berries
- 2 tbsp almond butter
- 1 tbsp maple syrup
- 1 tbsp chopped nuts (such as almonds or walnuts)

Preparation:

Combine cooked quinoa and mixed berries in a bowl.

Drizzle with almond butter and maple syrup.

Sprinkle with chopped nuts before serving.

## 2.  Chia Seed Pudding

Ingredients:

- 2 tbsp chia seeds
- 1/2 cup almond milk
- 1/2 tsp vanilla extract
- 1 tbsp maple syrup
- Fresh fruit for topping

Preparation:

In a bowl, mix chia seeds, almond milk, vanilla extract, and maple syrup.

Let it sit for at least 30 minutes or overnight in the refrigerator until thickened.

Serve topped with fresh fruit.

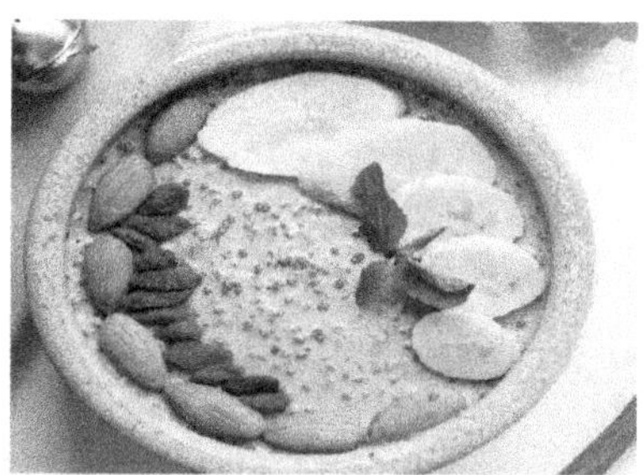

3.  Vegan Pancakes

Ingredients:

- 1 cup gluten-free flour blend
- 1 tbsp ground flaxseed + 3 tbsp water (flax egg)
- 1 cup almond milk
- 2 tbsp maple syrup
- 1 tsp baking powder
- 1/2 tsp vanilla extract
- Pinch of salt

Preparation:

In a bowl, whisk together the flax egg, almond milk, maple syrup, and vanilla extract.

Stir in the gluten-free flour blend, baking powder, and salt until well combined.

Heat a non-stick skillet over medium heat and pour batter into the skillet to form pancakes.

Cook until surface bubbles appear, then turn and continue cooking until both sides are golden brown.

Top with your preferred ingredients, such as maple syrup, nut butter, or fresh fruit.

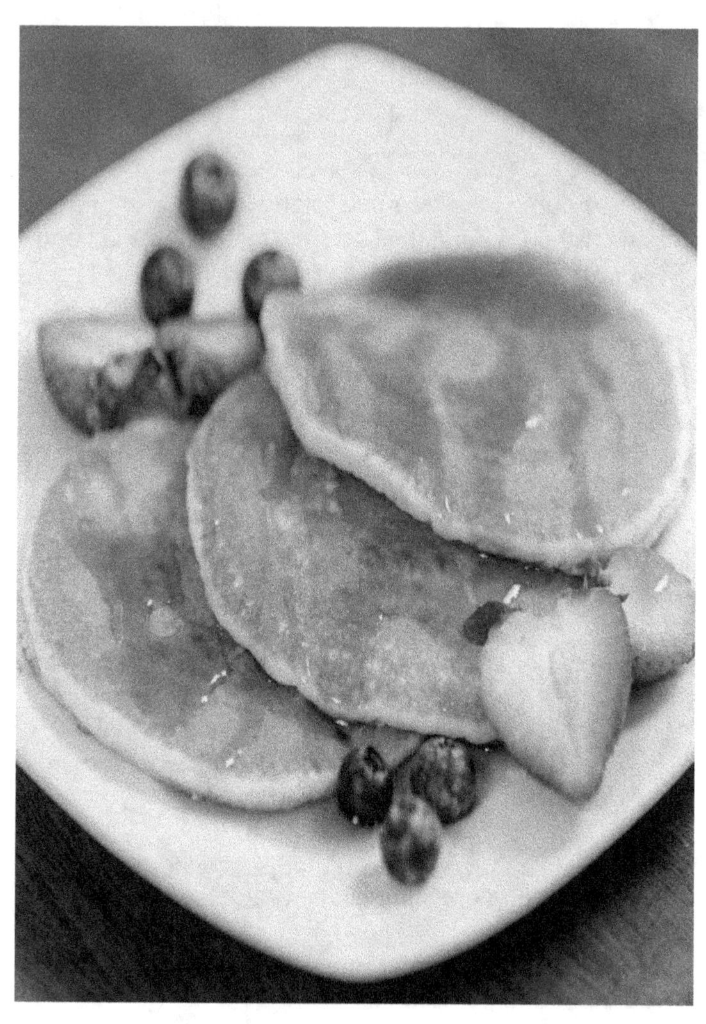

4.  Avocado Toast

Ingredients:

- 2 slices gluten-free bread, toasted
- 1 ripe avocado
- 1 tsp lemon juice
- Salt and pepper to taste

Optional toppings: sliced tomatoes, microgreens, red pepper flakes

Preparation:

In a small bowl, mash the avocado with lemon juice, salt, and pepper.

Spread the mashed avocado evenly on toasted gluten-free bread slices.

Top with your favorite toppings and serve immediately.

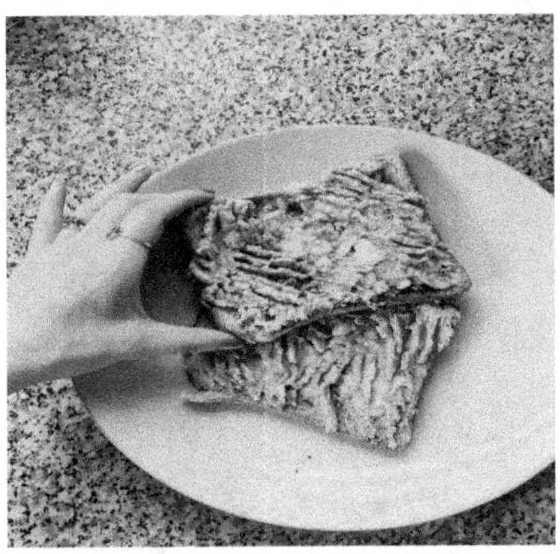

## 5. Tofu Scramble

Ingredients:

- 200g firm tofu, crumbled
- 1/4 cup diced onion
- 1/4 cup diced bell pepper
- 1/4 cup diced tomato
- 1/2 tsp turmeric powder
- 1/2 tsp garlic powder
- Salt and pepper to taste
- Fresh parsley for garnish

Preparation:

Heat a skillet over medium heat and sauté onion and bell pepper until softened.

Add crumbled tofu, turmeric powder, garlic powder, salt, and pepper. Cook until tofu is heated through and lightly browned.

Stir in diced tomatoes and cook for another minute.

Garnish with fresh parsley before serving.

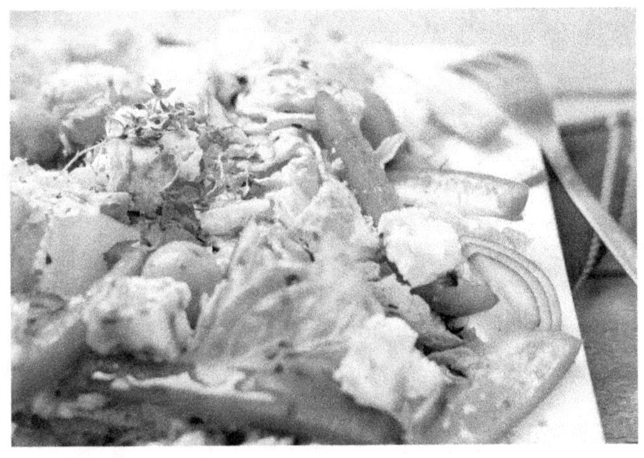

## 6. Coconut Yogurt Parfait

Ingredients:

- 1 cup coconut yogurt
- 1/4 cup gluten-free granola
- 1/4 cup mixed berries
- 1 tbsp shredded coconut

Preparation:

In a glass or jar, layer coconut yogurt, gluten-free granola, and mixed berries.

Repeat the layers until the jar is filled.

Top with shredded coconut before serving.

## 7. Smoothie Bowl

Ingredients:

- 1 frozen banana
- 1/2 cup frozen mixed berries
- 1/2 cup almond milk
- 2 tbsp gluten-free rolled oats

Toppings: sliced banana, granola, chia seeds and shredded coconut.

Preparation:

In a blender, combine frozen banana, frozen mixed berries, almond milk, and rolled oats.

Blend until smooth and creamy.

Pour into a bowl and add desired toppings before serving.

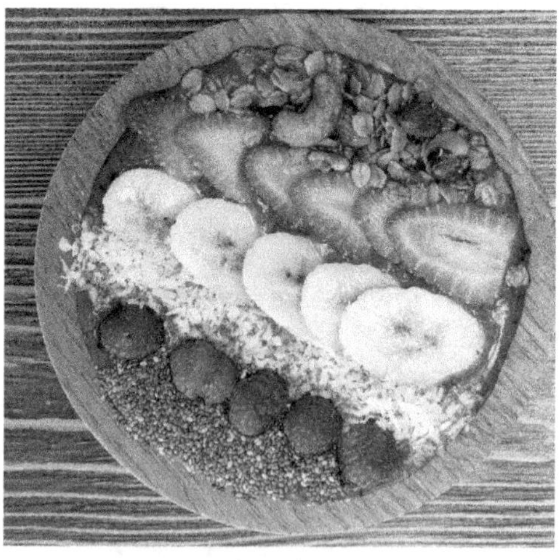

8.  Sweet Potato Breakfast Hash

Ingredients:

- 1 medium sweet potato, diced
- 1/4 cup diced onion
- 1/4 cup diced bell pepper
- 1/4 cup black beans, drained and rinsed
- 1/2 tsp smoked paprika
- Salt and pepper to taste
- Fresh cilantro for garnish

Preparation:

Heat a skillet over medium heat and sauté sweet potato, onion, and bell pepper until sweet potato is tender.

Add black beans, smoked paprika, salt, and pepper. Cook for another 2-3 minutes.

Garnish with fresh cilantro before serving.

9.  Banana Walnut Muffins

Ingredients:

- 1 cup mashed ripe banana
- 1/4 cup maple syrup
- 1/4 cup almond milk
- 2 tbsp coconut oil, melted
- 1 tsp vanilla extract
- 1 1/2 cups gluten-free flour blend
- 1 tsp baking powder
- 1/2 tsp baking soda
- 1/4 tsp salt
- 1/2 cup chopped walnuts

Preparation:

Grease a muffin tin with cooking spray and preheat the oven to 350°F (175°C).

In a large bowl, whisk together mashed banana, maple syrup, almond milk, coconut oil, and vanilla extract.

Stir in gluten-free flour blend, baking powder, baking soda, and salt until just combined.

Fold in chopped walnuts.

Once a toothpick inserted into the center comes out clean, bake the muffins for 20 to 25 minutes, dividing the batter equally among the cups.

Allow muffins to cool before serving.

## 10.  Tropical Smoothie

Ingredients:

- 1 cup frozen mango chunks
- 1/2 cup frozen pineapple chunks
- 1 ripe banana
- 1/2 cup coconut water
- 1/2 cup almond milk
- Optional add-ins: spinach, kale, chia seeds, protein powder

Preparation:

In a blender, combine frozen mango chunks, frozen pineapple chunks, ripe banana, coconut water, and almond milk.

Blend until smooth and creamy.

Add optional add-ins if desired and blend again until well combined.

Pour into glasses and serve immediately.

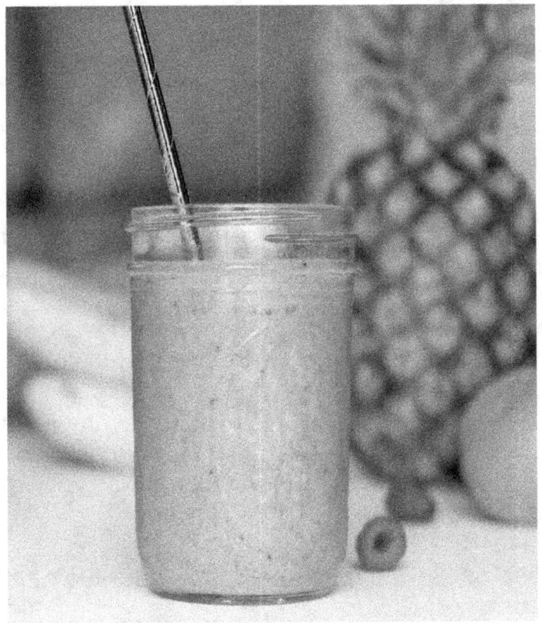

## 11.  Cinnamon-Cherry Oatmeal

Ingredients:

- 1 cup gluten-free rolled oats
- 2 cups water
- 1/2 cup cherries, pitted and halved
- 1/2 teaspoon ground cinnamon
- Two tablespoons of your preferred sweetener, or maple syrup
- Pinch of salt
- Optional toppings: sliced almonds, coconut flakes, additional cherries

Preparation:

Heat a saucepan over medium-high heat and bring the water to a boil.

Once the water is boiling, add the rolled oats, cherries, ground cinnamon, maple syrup, and a pinch of salt.

Reduce the heat to low and simmer, stirring occasionally, for about 5-7 minutes, or until the oats are tender and the mixture has thickened to your desired consistency.

Take the saucepan off of the burner after the oatmeal is cooked.

Serve the cinnamon-cherry oatmeal hot, portioned into bowls.

Garnish with optional toppings such as sliced almonds, coconut flakes, and additional cherries if desired.

Enjoy your warm and comforting cinnamon-cherry oatmeal breakfast!

This recipe serves approximately 2 servings.You are welcome to change the amounts to suit your tastes and the quantity required for the number of servings.


## 12.   Kale and Pear Smoothie

Ingredients:

- 1 ripe pear, cored and chopped
- 1 cup kale leaves, stems removed
- 1/2 banana
- 1/2 cup plant-based milk, such as almond milk
- 1/2 cup plain dairy-free yogurt
- 1 tablespoon honey or maple syrup (optional, for sweetness)
- Ice cubes (optional)

Preparation:

Place all ingredients in a blender.

Blend until smooth and creamy, adding more almond milk if necessary to reach your desired consistency.

Taste and adjust sweetness if needed by adding honey or maple syrup.

Pour into glasses and serve immediately.

## 13.  Banana and Spinach Smoothie

Ingredients:

- 1 ripe banana
- 1 cup fresh spinach leaves
- 1/2 cup frozen pineapple chunks
- 1/2 cup plant-based milk (like Almond milk)
- 1 tablespoon chia seeds (optional, for added nutrition)
- Ice cubes (optional)

Preparation:

In a blender, combine the banana, spinach, frozen pineapple chunks, almond milk, and chia seeds.

Blend until smooth and creamy.
If the smoothie is too thick, add more almond milk as needed to reach your desired consistency.

Pour into glasses and serve immediately.

## 14.  Oat and Raspberry Crepes

Ingredients for Crepes:

- 1 cup gluten-free flour
- 1/4 cup rolled oats
- 1 cup almond milk (or any plant-based milk)
- 2 tablespoons melted coconut oil (or vegan butter)
- 1 tablespoon maple syrup
- 1 teaspoon vanilla extract
- Pinch of salt

Ingredients for Filling:

- 1 cup fresh raspberries
- 1 tablespoon maple syrup (optional, for added sweetness)
- Vegan yogurt or whipped coconut cream (optional, for serving)

Preparation:

In a mixing bowl, whisk together the gluten-free flour, rolled oats, almond milk, melted coconut oil, maple syrup, vanilla extract, and a pinch of salt until smooth.

Grease a non-stick skillet with coconut oil and heat it over medium heat.

Pour a small amount of the crepe batter into the skillet, swirling to spread evenly.

Cook for one to two minutes, or until the bottom is lightly golden and the edges are beginning to lift.

The crepe should be cooked for a further one to two minutes after being carefully flipped.

Repeat with the remaining batter.

In a separate bowl, gently mash the fresh raspberries with maple syrup, if using, to create a compote.

To assemble, spread a spoonful of the raspberry compote onto each crepe and fold or roll it up.

Serve warm with a dollop of vegan yogurt or whipped coconut cream if desired.

## 15.  Cauliflower Hash Browns

Ingredients:

- 1 small head cauliflower, grated
- 1/4 cup gluten-free breadcrumbs
- 2 tablespoons nutritional yeast
- 1 teaspoon garlic powder
- 1 teaspoon onion powder
- Salt and pepper to taste
- Olive oil for cooking

Preparation:

In a large mixing bowl, combine the grated cauliflower, gluten-free breadcrumbs, nutritional yeast, garlic powder, onion powder, salt, and pepper. Mix until well combined.

Pour some olive oil into a skillet and heat it over medium heat.

Form the cauliflower mixture into patties and place them in the skillet.

Cook for 4-5 minutes on each side, or until golden brown and crispy.

Remove from the skillet and drain on a paper towel-lined plate.

Serve hot as a side dish or breakfast hash.

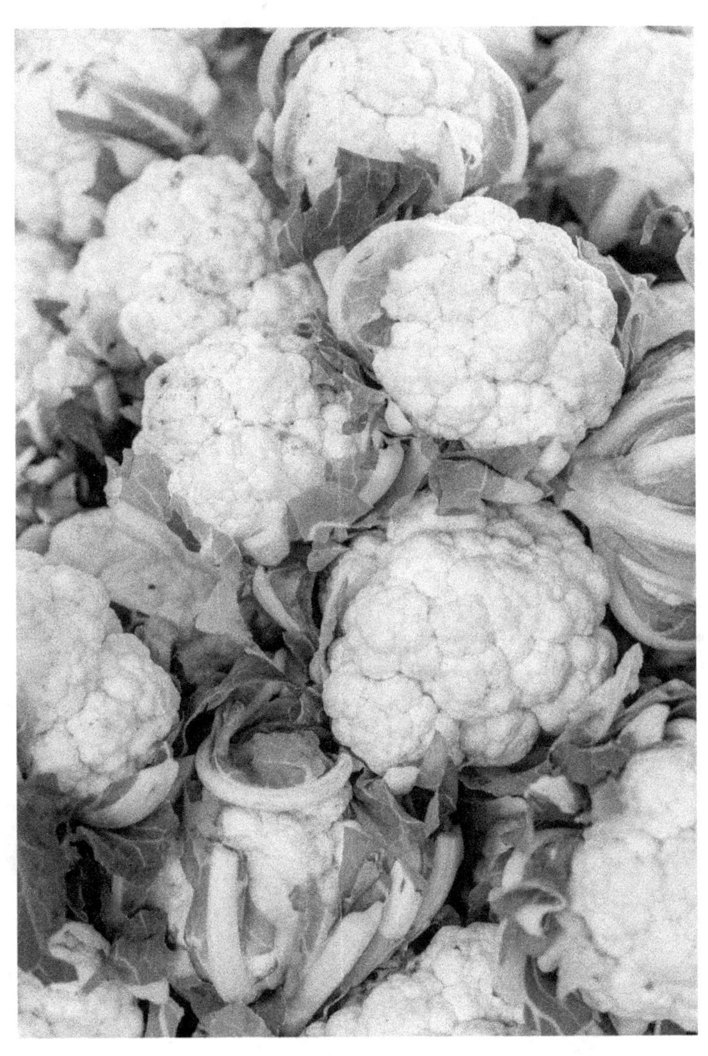

16. scrambled eggs and salmon (using plant-based alternatives)

Ingredients:

For the Vegan Scrambled Eggs:

- 1 block (14 oz) firm tofu,  pressed and drained.
- 2 tablespoons nutritional yeast
- 1 tablespoon olive oil
- 1/2 teaspoon ground turmeric (for color)
- Salt and pepper to taste
- Optional: chopped vegetables (such as bell peppers, onions, spinach)

For the "Salmon":

- 1 can (14 oz) hearts of palm, drained and chopped into small pieces
- 1 tablespoon tamari (Gluten-free alternative for Soy sauce)
- 1 tablespoon liquid smoke
- 1 tablespoon olive oil
- Salt and pepper to taste

For Serving:

- Gluten-free toast or English muffins
- Sliced avocado
- Fresh herbs (such as parsley or chives)

Preparation:

Prepare the Vegan Scrambled Eggs:

In a mixing bowl, crumble the drained tofu with your hands or a fork

Add nutritional yeast, olive oil, ground turmeric, salt, and pepper to the crumbled tofu. Mix well to combine.

Heat a non-stick skillet over medium heat. Add the tofu mixture to the skillet and cook for 5-7 minutes, stirring occasionally, until heated through and slightly golden. If using chopped vegetables, add them to the skillet and cook until tender.

Once cooked, remove the vegan scrambled eggs from heat and set aside.

Prepare the "Salmon":

In a separate mixing bowl, combine the chopped hearts of palm, soy sauce or tamari, liquid smoke, olive oil, salt, and pepper. Toss until well coated.

Heat a non-stick skillet over medium-high heat. Add the marinated hearts of palm to the skillet and cook for 5-7 minutes, stirring occasionally, until lightly browned and slightly crispy.

Once cooked, remove the "salmon" from heat and set aside.

Assemble the Dish:

Toast gluten-free bread slices or English muffins until golden brown.

Spread a generous portion of the vegan scrambled eggs on each toast or English muffin.

Top the scrambled eggs with a serving of the "salmon" hearts of palm.

Garnish with sliced avocado and fresh herbs.

Serve immediately and enjoy your gluten-free vegan scrambled eggs and "salmon" for a delicious and satisfying meal!

This recipe provides a plant-based alternative to traditional scrambled eggs and salmon, offering a flavorful and protein-rich dish suitable for those following a gluten-free and vegan lifestyle.

## 17. Lemon French Toasts

Ingredients:

- 4 slices of gluten-free bread
- 2 tablespoons lemon juice
- Zest of 1 lemon
- 1/2 cup almond milk (or any plant-based milk)
- 2 tablespoons chickpea flour (or any gluten-free flour)
- 1 tablespoon maple syrup
- 1/2 teaspoon vanilla extract
- Pinch of salt
- Coconut oil or vegan butter for cooking

Preparation:

In a shallow dish, whisk together the lemon juice, lemon zest, almond milk, chickpea flour, maple syrup, vanilla extract, and salt until well combined.

Heat a drizzle of coconut oil or vegan butter in a skillet over medium heat.

Dip each slice of gluten-free bread into the lemon mixture, ensuring both sides are coated evenly.

Place the coated bread slices in the skillet and cook for 2-3 minutes on each side, or until golden brown and crispy.

Remove from the skillet and serve hot with your favorite toppings such as fresh berries, maple syrup, or vegan whipped cream.

18.  Coconut French toast:

Ingredients:

- 4 slices of gluten-free vegan bread (such as almond flour bread or coconut flour bread)
- 1/2 cup full-fat coconut milk
- 2 tablespoons chickpea flour (also known as besan or gram flour)
- 1 tablespoon maple syrup or agave syrup
- 1/2 teaspoon ground cinnamon
- 1/2 teaspoon vanilla extract
- Pinch of salt
- Coconut oil or vegan butter for cooking
- Optional toppings: sliced fruits, shredded coconut, maple syrup, dairy-free yogurt

Preparation:

In a shallow dish or bowl, whisk together the coconut milk, chickpea flour, maple syrup or agave syrup, ground cinnamon, vanilla extract, and a pinch of salt until smooth and well combined.

Heat a non-stick skillet or frying pan over medium heat and add a little coconut oil or vegan butter to grease the surface.

Dip each slice of gluten-free vegan bread into the coconut milk mixture, ensuring both sides are coated evenly.

Place the soaked bread slices onto the preheated skillet and cook for 3-4 minutes on each side, or until golden brown and crispy.

Repeat with the remaining slices of bread, adding more coconut oil or vegan butter to the skillet as needed.

Once all the French toast slices are cooked, transfer them to serving plates.

Serve the gluten-free vegan coconut French toast warm, topped with your favorite toppings such as sliced fruits, shredded coconut, maple syrup, or dairy-free yogurt.

Enjoy your delicious and indulgent gluten-free vegan coconut French toast for a satisfying breakfast or brunch!

This recipe offers a tropical twist to traditional French toast, thanks to the coconut milk and shredded coconut. It's perfect for anyone following a gluten-free and vegan lifestyle!

## 19. Blueberry Ginger Smoothie:

Ingredients:

- 1 cup frozen blueberries
- 1 ripe banana
- 1/2 cup non-dairy milk (such as almond milk, coconut milk, or soy milk)
- 1/2 cup dairy-free yogurt (such as coconut yogurt or almond yogurt)

- 1 tablespoon fresh ginger, grated
- 1 tablespoon maple syrup or agave syrup (optional, adjust to taste)
- 1 tablespoon chia seeds (optional, for added thickness and nutrition)
- Ice cubes (optional, for a colder smoothie)

Preparation:

In the specified order, put all of the ingredients into a blender.

Blend on high speed until smooth and creamy. If the smoothie is too thick, you can add more non-dairy milk to reach your desired consistency.

Taste the smoothie and adjust sweetness if needed by adding more maple syrup or agave syrup.

Once the smoothie is blended to your liking, pour it into glasses.

Optionally, garnish with a few fresh blueberries or a slice of ginger.

Serve immediately and enjoy your refreshing and nutritious gluten-free vegan Blueberry Ginger Smoothie!

This smoothie is packed with antioxidants from the blueberries, and the addition of fresh ginger adds a refreshing zing and anti-inflammatory properties. It's a perfect way to start your day or as a midday pick-me-up!

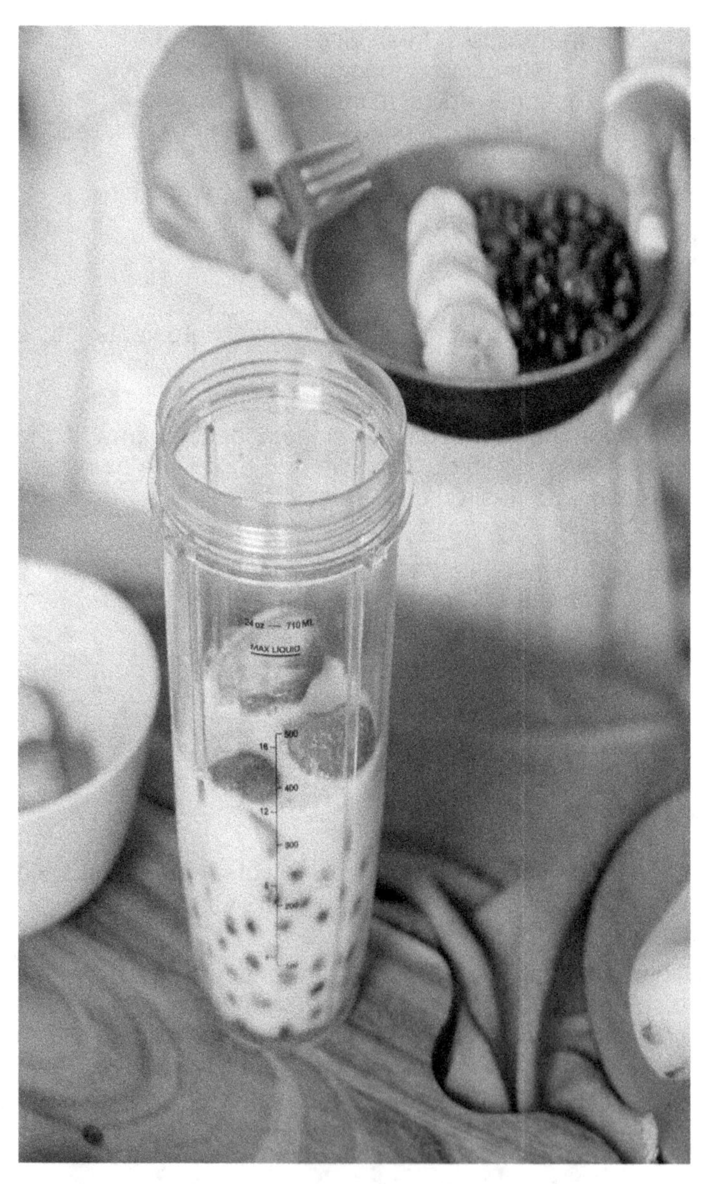

20.  Coconut flour pancakes:

Ingredients:

- 1/2 cup coconut flour
- 2 tablespoons ground flaxseed meal
- 6 tablespoons water
- 1 cup non-dairy milk (such as almond milk, coconut milk, or soy milk)
- 2 tablespoons maple syrup or agave syrup
- 1 teaspoon baking powder
- 1/2 teaspoon vanilla extract
- Pinch of salt
- Coconut oil or vegan butter for cooking

Optional toppings:

- Sliced fruits (such as, berries, bananas or peaches)
- Maple syrup or agave syrup
- Coconut flakes
- Chopped nuts or seeds

Preparation:

Mix together, in a small bowl, the ground flaxseed meal and water. Let it sit for about 5 minutes to thicken and form a flax "egg".

In a mixing bowl, combine the coconut flour, flax "egg", non-dairy milk, maple syrup or agave syrup, baking powder, vanilla extract, and a pinch of salt. Mix thoroughly until a smooth batter is formed. To enable the coconut flour to absorb the liquid, let the batter sit for a few minutes.

Over medium heat, preheat a nonstick skillet or griddle.. Add a small amount of coconut oil or vegan butter to the skillet and let it melt.

To make pancakes the size you want, pour some of the batter onto the skillet.

Cook for 2 to 3 minutes, or until the edges begin to set and bubbles appear on the surface of the pancakes.

Carefully flip the pancakes and cook for an additional 1-2 minutes on the other side, or until golden brown and cooked through.

Repeat with the remaining batter, adding more coconut oil or vegan butter to the skillet as needed.

Serve the gluten-free vegan coconut flour pancakes warm, topped with your favorite toppings such as sliced fruits, maple syrup or agave syrup, coconut flakes, chopped nuts or seeds.

Enjoy your delicious and fluffy gluten-free vegan coconut flour pancakes for a satisfying breakfast or brunch!


21.  Gluten-Free Vegan Oatmeal

Ingredients:

- 1 cup gluten-free rolled oats
- 2 cups water or non-dairy milk (such as almond milk, coconut milk, or soy milk)
- Pinch of salt
- Optional toppings: sliced fruits (such as bananas, berries, or apples), nuts (such as almonds, walnuts, or pecans), seeds (such as

chia seeds or pumpkin seeds), maple syrup or agave syrup, cinnamon, coconut flakes

Preparation:

In a small saucepan, combine the gluten-free rolled oats and water (or non-dairy milk) over medium heat.

Add a pinch of salt to the mixture. Stir well to combine.

After bringing the mixture to a gentle boil, turn down the heat.

Let the oatmeal simmer, stirring occasionally, for about 5-7 minutes or until the oats are cooked and the mixture has thickened to your desired consistency. If you prefer a creamier texture, you can cook it for a little longer.

Once the oatmeal is ready, remove it from the heat and let it cool slightly.

Serve the gluten-free vegan oatmeal warm, topped with your favorite toppings such as sliced fruits, nuts, seeds, maple syrup or agave syrup, cinnamon, or coconut flakes.

Enjoy your delicious and nutritious gluten-free vegan oatmeal for a comforting breakfast!

This oatmeal recipe is customizable, so feel free to experiment with different toppings and flavors to suit your taste preferences. It's a hearty and wholesome breakfast option that will keep you full and satisfied until lunchtime.

22.  Banana pancakes:

Ingredients:

- 1 ripe banana
- 1 cup gluten-free oat flour (you can make this by blending gluten-free rolled oats in a food processor until finely ground)
- 1 tablespoon ground flaxseed meal
- 2 tablespoons water
- 1/2 cup non-dairy milk (such as almond milk, coconut milk, or soy milk)
- 1 teaspoon baking powder
- 1/2 teaspoon vanilla extract
- Pinch of salt
- Coconut oil or vegan butter for cooking

Optional toppings:

- Sliced bananas
- Berries
- Maple syrup or agave syrup
- Nut butter
- Chopped nuts or seeds

Preparation:

In a small bowl, mix together the ground flaxseed meal and water. Let it sit for about 5 minutes to thicken and form a flax "egg".

Mash the ripe banana with a fork in a mixing bowl until smooth.

Add the gluten-free oat flour, flax "egg", non-dairy milk, baking powder, vanilla extract, and a pinch of salt to the mashed banana. Mix thoroughly until a smooth batter is formed. You can thin out the batter by adding a little extra non-dairy milk if it's too thick.

On medium heat, preheat a nonstick skillet or griddle. heat. Add a small amount of coconut oil or vegan butter to the skillet and let it melt.

Pour a portion of the pancake batter into the skillet to make pancakes of your desired size.

Cook the pancakes for 2-3 minutes, until bubbles appear on the surface and the edges begin to set.

Carefully flip the pancakes and cook for an additional 1-2 minutes on the other side, or until golden brown and cooked through.

Continue with the remaining batter, adjusting the skillet's oil content with more coconut oil or vegan butter as needed.

Serve the gluten-free vegan banana pancakes warm, topped with your favorite toppings such as sliced bananas, berries, maple syrup or agave syrup, nut butter, chopped nuts or seeds.

Enjoy your delicious and fluffy gluten-free vegan banana pancakes for a satisfying breakfast or brunch!

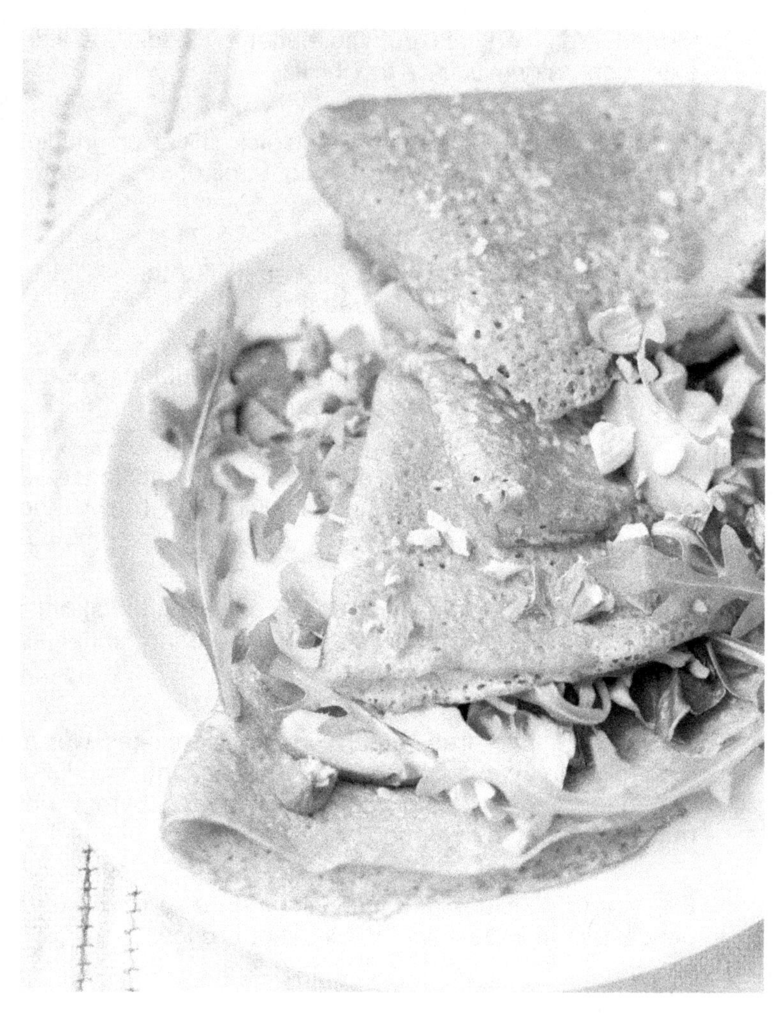

23.  Quinoa Cinnamon Orange Porridge:

Ingredients:

- 1 cup cooked quinoa
- 1 cup unsweetened almond milk (or any other plant-based milk)
- 1 orange (juice and zest)
- 2 tablespoons maple syrup or agave syrup
- 1 teaspoon ground cinnamon
- 1/4 teaspoon ground nutmeg
- Pinch of salt
- Optional toppings: sliced oranges, chopped nuts, seeds, coconut flakes

Preparation:

In a saucepan, combine the cooked quinoa and almond milk over medium heat.

Zest the orange using a zester or grater, then juice the orange. Add the orange zest and juice to the saucepan.

Stir in the maple syrup (or agave syrup), ground cinnamon, ground nutmeg, and a pinch of salt.

Cook the mixture, stirring occasionally, until it comes to a gentle simmer. Reduce the heat to low and let it simmer for about 5-7 minutes, or until the porridge thickens to your desired consistency.

Once the porridge is ready, remove it from the heat and let it cool slightly.

Serve the gluten-free vegan quinoa cinnamon orange porridge warm, topped with sliced oranges, chopped nuts, seeds, coconut flakes, or any other desired toppings.

Enjoy your comforting and nutritious quinoa cinnamon orange porridge for a delicious breakfast or snack!

This porridge is not only gluten-free and vegan but also packed with protein, fiber, and vitamins from the quinoa and oranges. It's an excellent way to start your day on a healthy note.


## 24.  Oatmeal Banana Date Waffles

Ingredients:

- 1 cup gluten-free rolled oats
- 2 ripe bananas
- 1/4 cup chopped dates
- 2 tablespoons ground flaxseed meal
- 6 tablespoons water
- 1/4 cup non-dairy milk (such as almond milk, coconut milk, or soy milk)
- 2 tablespoons coconut oil, melted (plus extra for greasing the waffle iron)
- 1 teaspoon baking powder
- 1/2 teaspoon vanilla extract
- Pinch of salt

Optional toppings:

- Sliced bananas
- Chopped dates
- Maple syrup
- Dairy-free yogurt
- Chopped nuts or seeds

Preparation:

Preheat your waffle iron according to the manufacturer's instructions.

In a small bowl, mix together the ground flaxseed meal and water. Let it sit for about 5 minutes to thicken and form a flax "egg".

In a blender or food processor, combine the gluten-free rolled oats, ripe bananas, chopped dates, flax "egg", non-dairy milk, melted coconut oil, baking powder, vanilla extract, and a pinch of salt.

Blend the ingredients until smooth and well combined. The batter should have a thick, pourable consistency. If it's too thick, you can add a little more non-dairy milk to thin it out.

Once the waffle iron is heated, lightly grease the surface with coconut oil or non-stick spray.

Pour enough batter onto the center of the waffle iron to cover about two-thirds of the surface area (the batter will expand when cooked).

Close the waffle iron and cook according to the manufacturer's instructions, until the waffles are golden brown and crispy.

Carefully remove the waffles from the iron and transfer them to a plate.

Serve the gluten-free vegan oatmeal banana date waffles warm, topped with sliced bananas, chopped dates, maple syrup, dairy-free yogurt, chopped nuts or seeds, or any other desired toppings.

Enjoy your delicious and nutritious gluten-free vegan oatmeal banana date waffles for breakfast or brunch!


## 25. Quinoa and Oat Waffles

Ingredients:

- 1 cup cooked quinoa
- 1 cup gluten-free rolled oats
- 1 ripe banana
- 2 tablespoons ground flaxseed meal
- 6 tablespoons water
- 1/4 cup non-dairy milk (such as almond milk, coconut milk, or soy milk)
- 2 tablespoons coconut oil, melted (plus extra for greasing the waffle iron)
- 1 teaspoon baking powder
- 1/2 teaspoon vanilla extract
- Pinch of salt
- Optional: maple syrup or fruit compote for serving
- Optional toppings: fresh fruits, nuts, seeds, dairy-free yogurt

Preparation:

As directed by the manufacturer, preheat your waffle iron.

Combine the water and ground flaxseed meal in a small bowl.. Let it sit for about 5 minutes to thicken and form a flax "egg".

In a blender or food processor, combine the cooked quinoa, gluten-free rolled oats, ripe banana, flax "egg", non-dairy milk, melted coconut oil, baking powder, vanilla extract, and a pinch of salt.

Blend the ingredients until smooth and well combined. The batter should have a pourable, thick consistency. If it's too thick, you can add a little more non-dairy milk to thin it out.

Once the waffle iron is heated, lightly grease the surface with coconut oil or non-stick spray.

Pour enough batter onto the center of the waffle iron to cover about two-thirds of the surface area (the batter will expand when cooked).

Close the waffle iron and cook according to the manufacturer's instructions, until the waffles are golden brown and crispy.

Remove the waffles carefully from the iron and place them on a plate. Repeat with the remaining batter.

Serve the gluten-free vegan quinoa and oat waffles warm, with your choice of toppings such as maple syrup or fruit compote, fresh fruits, nuts, seeds, or dairy-free yogurt.

Enjoy your delicious and nutritious gluten-free vegan quinoa and oat waffles for breakfast!

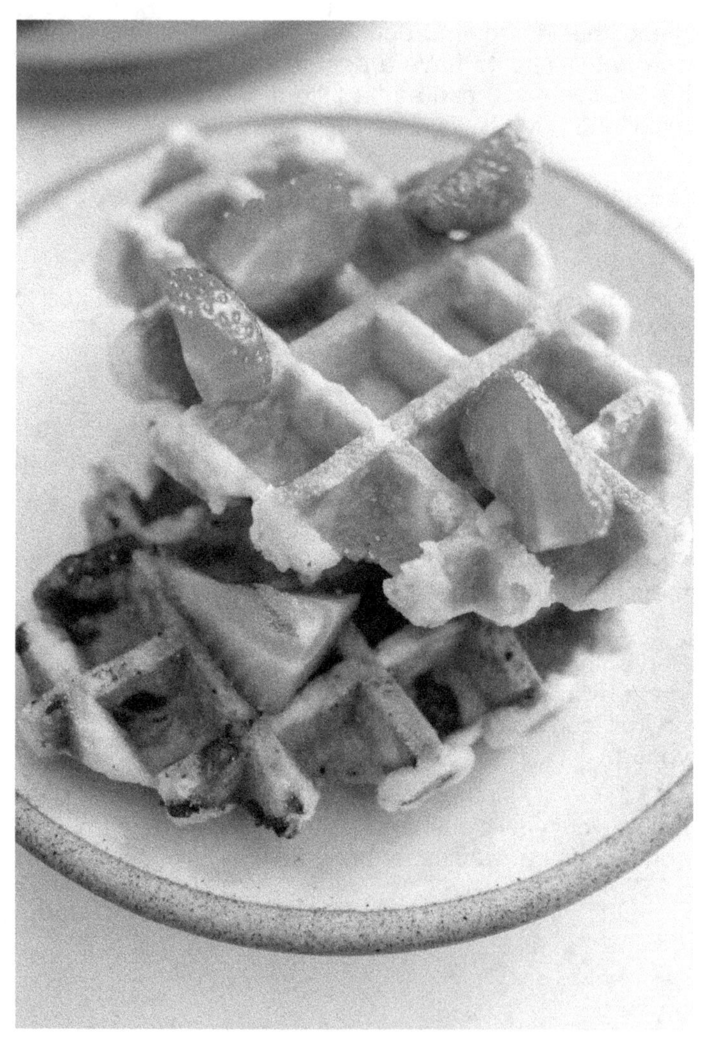

## 1. Quinoa Salad with Roasted Vegetables

Ingredients:

- 1 cup quinoa
- Assorted vegetables, including cherry tomatoes, zucchini, and bell peppers
- Olive oil
- Salt and pepper
- Lemon juice
- Fresh herbs (such as parsley or basil)

Preparation:

Cook quinoa according to package instructions.

Chop vegetables into bite-sized pieces and toss with olive oil, salt, and pepper.

Roast vegetables in the oven at 400°F (200°C) for 20-25 minutes until tender and slightly charred.

Mix cooked quinoa with roasted vegetables. Add lemon juice and fresh herbs for extra flavor. Serve warm or chilled.

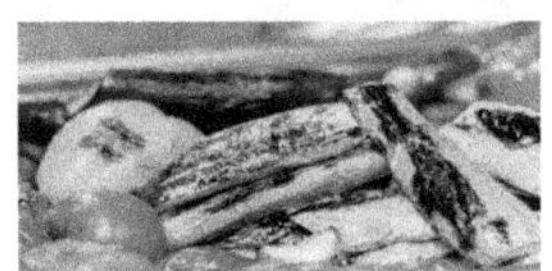

2. Vegan Lentil Soup

Ingredients:

- 1 cup dried lentils
- Assorted vegetables (such as carrots, celery, onions)
- Vegetable broth
- Garlic
- Bay leaves
- Salt and pepper
- Fresh parsley (for garnish)

Preparation:

Rinse lentils under cold water and drain.

Chop vegetables and mince garlic.

In a large pot, sauté vegetables and garlic until softened.

Add lentils, vegetable broth, bay leaves, salt, and pepper. Bring to a boil, then reduce heat and simmer for 20-25 minutes until lentils are tender.

Remove bay leaves and adjust seasoning if necessary. Serve hot, garnished with fresh parsley.

## 3. Chickpea and Avocado Wrap

Ingredients:

- Gluten-free wraps or tortillas
- Canned chickpeas
- Avocado
- Mixed greens
- Cherry tomatoes
- Tahini or hummus
- Lemon juice
- Salt and pepper

Preparation:

Rinse and drain chickpeas. Mash them in a bowl with avocado, lemon juice, salt, and pepper.

Spread tahini or hummus on gluten-free wraps.

Layer mashed chickpea and avocado mixture, mixed greens, and sliced cherry tomatoes on top of the wrap.

Roll up tightly and slice in half. Serve immediately or pack for a to-go lunch.

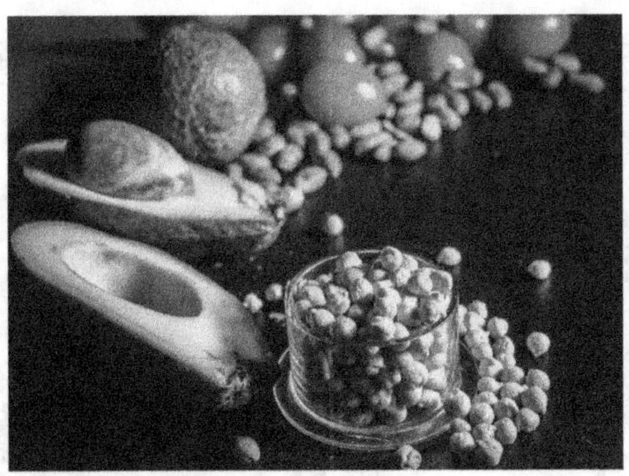

4.  Sweet Potato and Black Beans Salad

Ingredients:

- Roasted sweet potatoes
- Cooked black beans
- Red onion
- Bell peppers
- Lime juice
- Cilantro
- Cumin
- Salt and pepper

Preparation:

Cube and roast sweet potatoes in the oven until tender.

Rinse and drain black beans. Chop red onion and bell peppers.

In a large bowl, combine roasted sweet potatoes, black beans, red onion, and bell peppers.

Dress with lime juice, chopped cilantro, cumin, salt, and pepper. Toss to combine. Serve as a hearty salad.

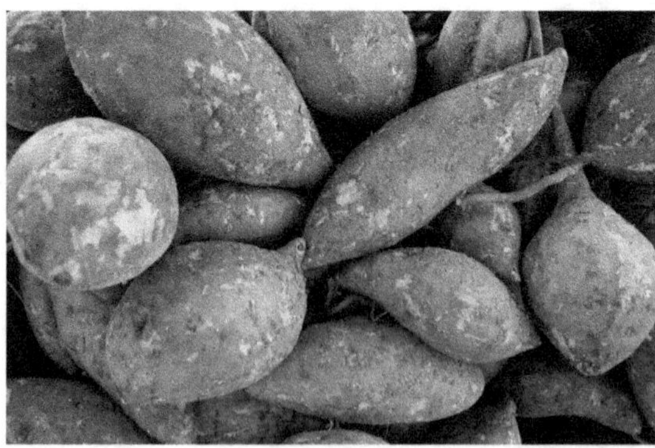

## 5.  Quinoa Stuffed Bell Peppers

Ingredients:

- Bell peppers
- Cooked quinoa
- Canned black beans
- Corn kernels
- Diced tomatoes
- Onion
- Garlic
- Cumin
- Chili powder
- Salt and pepper

Preparation:

Preheat the oven to 375°F (190°C). Cut tops off bell peppers and remove seeds and membranes.

In a skillet, sauté onion and garlic until softened. Add diced tomatoes, black beans, corn kernels, cooked quinoa, cumin, chili powder, salt, and pepper. Cook until heated through.

Stuff bell peppers with quinoa mixture and place in a baking dish.

Bake for 25-30 minutes until bell peppers are tender. Serve hot.

## 6.  Chickpea Salad Sandwich

Ingredients:

- Canned chickpeas
- Celery
- Red onion
- Vegan mayo
- Dijon mustard
- Lemon juice
- Salt and pepper
- Lettuce
- Gluten-free bread

Preparation:

Rinse and drain chickpeas. In a bowl, mash them with a fork or potato masher.

Finely chop celery and red onion. Add to  the mashed chickpeas.

Mix in vegan mayo, Dijon mustard, lemon juice, salt, and pepper.

Toast gluten-free bread slices. Spread chickpea salad on bread and top with lettuce. Serve as a sandwich.

7.  Thai Peanut Noodles

Ingredients:

- Gluten-free rice noodles
- Broccoli
- Red bell pepper
- Carrots
- Green onions
- Peanut butter
- Soy sauce or tamari
- Lime juice
- Maple syrup
- Sriracha (optional)
- Crushed peanuts (for garnish)

Preparation:

Cook rice noodles according to package instructions. Drain and set aside.

Chop broccoli, red bell pepper, carrots, and green onions.

In a bowl, whisk together peanut butter, soy sauce or tamari, lime juice, maple syrup, and sriracha (if using) until smooth.

In a skillet, sauté chopped vegetables until tender.

Add cooked rice noodles and peanut sauce to the skillet. Toss until noodles are well coated and heated through.

Serve hot, garnished with crushed peanuts.

8.  Mediterranean Quinoa Bowl

Ingredients:

- Cooked quinoa
- Cherry tomatoes
- Cucumber
- Kalamata olives
- Red onion
- Fresh parsley
- Lemon juice
- Olive oil
- Salt and pepper
- Hummus
- Gluten-free falafel (optional)

Preparation:

Chop cherry tomatoes, cucumber, kalamata olives, and red onion.

In a bowl, combine cooked quinoa with chopped vegetables and fresh parsley.

Dress with lemon juice, olive oil, salt, and pepper. Toss to combine.

Serve quinoa salad in bowls with a dollop of hummus and gluten-free falafel if desired.

9.  Lentil Tacos

Ingredients:

- Cooked lentils
- Taco seasoning
- Corn tortillas
- Avocado
- Salsa
- Shredded lettuce
- Chopped tomatoes
- Lime wedges

Preparation:

In a skillet, heat cooked lentils with taco seasoning until heated through.

Warm corn tortillas in a dry skillet or microwave.

Assemble tacos by filling each tortilla with lentils, sliced avocado, salsa, shredded lettuce, and chopped tomatoes.

Serve with lime wedges for squeezing over tacos.

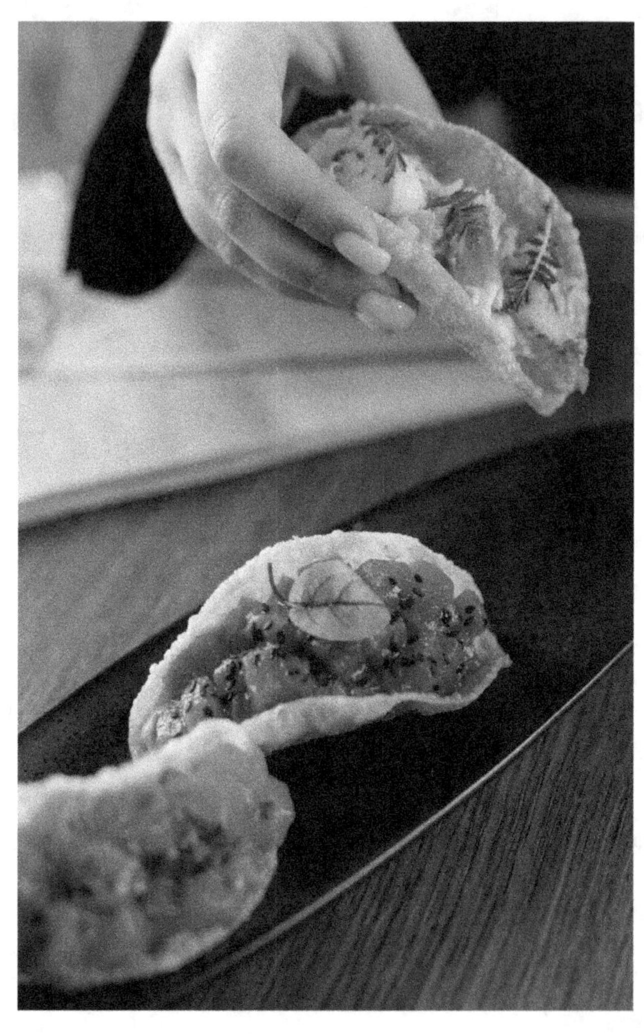

10.  Black Bean and Quinoa Burrito Bowl

Ingredients:

- Cooked quinoa
- Canned black beans
- Corn kernels
- Avocado
- Salsa
- Shredded lettuce
- Lime wedges
- Fresh cilantro

Preparation:

Rinse and drain black beans. Heat them in a skillet until heated through.

In bowls, layer cooked quinoa, black beans, corn kernels, sliced avocado, salsa, and shredded lettuce.

Garnish with lime wedges and fresh cilantro. Serve as a burrito bowl.

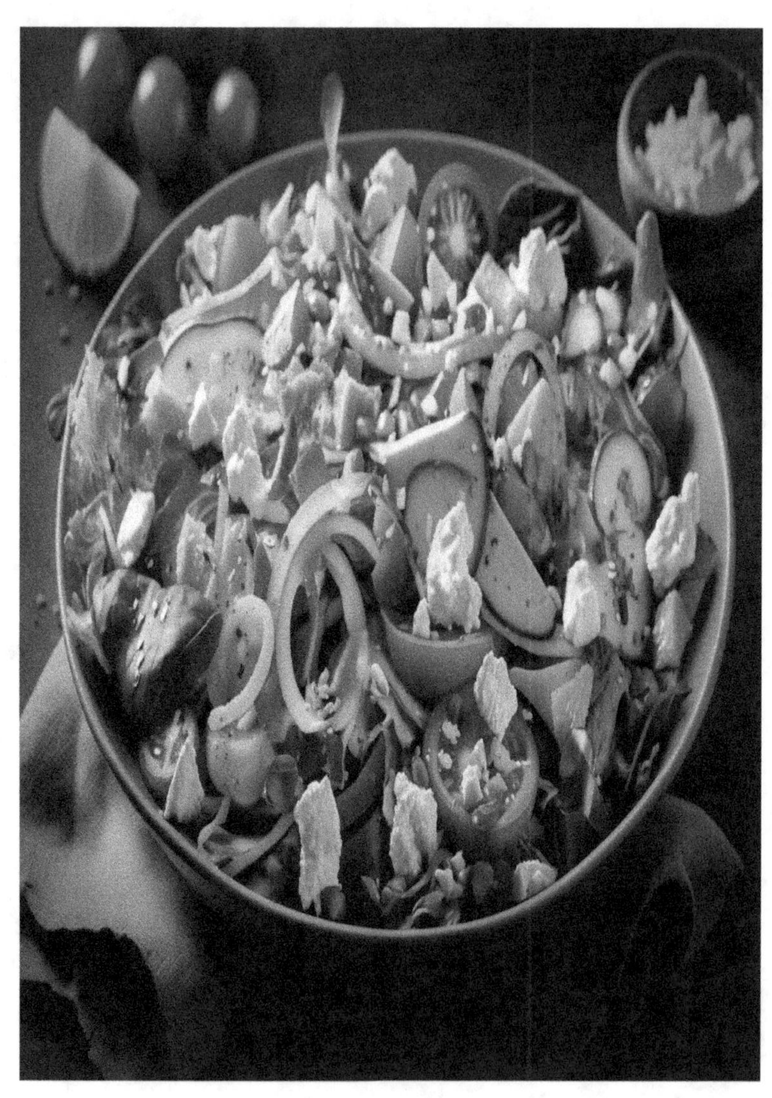

11.  Quinoa and Vegetable Stir-Fry:

Ingredients:

- 1 cup cooked quinoa
- Assorted vegetables (such as bell peppers, broccoli, carrots, snap peas)
- 2 tablespoons gluten-free tamari or soy sauce
- 1 tablespoon sesame oil
- 1 clove garlic, minced
- 1 teaspoon grated ginger
- Optional: tofu or tempeh for added protein

Preparation:

Heat Sesame oil over medium-high heat in a large skillet or wok.

Add the grated ginger and minced garlic, and cook for one minute.

Add assorted vegetables and cook until tender-crisp.

Stir in cooked quinoa and gluten-free tamari or soy sauce. Cook for an additional 2-3 minutes, stirring frequently.

Serve hot, optionally topped with cooked tofu or tempeh.

12.  Chickpea Salad Collard Wraps:

Ingredients:

- Collard green leaves (large)
- 1 can chickpeas, drained and rinsed
- 1/4 cup diced cucumber
- 1/4 cup diced red bell pepper
- 2 tablespoons diced red onion
- 2 tablespoons chopped fresh parsley
- 1 tablespoon lemon juice
- 1 tablespoon olive oil
- Salt and pepper to taste
- Hummus for spreading

Preparation:

In a mixing bowl, mash the chickpeas with a fork or potato masher.

Add diced cucumber, red bell pepper, red onion, parsley, lemon juice, olive oil, salt, and pepper to the mashed chickpeas. Mix well.

Place a collard green leaf flat on a plate. Spread a layer of hummus over the leaf.

Spoon the chickpea salad mixture onto the collard green leaf.

Fold the sides of the leaf inward and roll it up, creating a wrap.

Repeat with remaining collard green leaves and chickpea salad mixture.

Serve the wraps immediately or refrigerate for later.

13.  Mango and Black Bean Quinoa Salad:

Ingredients:

- 1 cup cooked quinoa
- 1 ripe mango, diced
- 1 can black beans, drained and rinsed
- 1/4 cup diced red onion
- 1/4 cup chopped fresh cilantro
- 2 tablespoons lime juice
- 1 tablespoon olive oil
- Salt and pepper to taste
- Optional: diced avocado for topping

Preparation:

In a large mixing bowl, combine cooked quinoa, diced mango, black beans, red onion, and chopped cilantro.

In a small bowl, whisk together lime juice, olive oil, salt, and pepper.

Pour the dressing over the quinoa salad mixture and toss until well combined.

Serve the salad at room temperature or chilled, optionally topped with diced avocado.

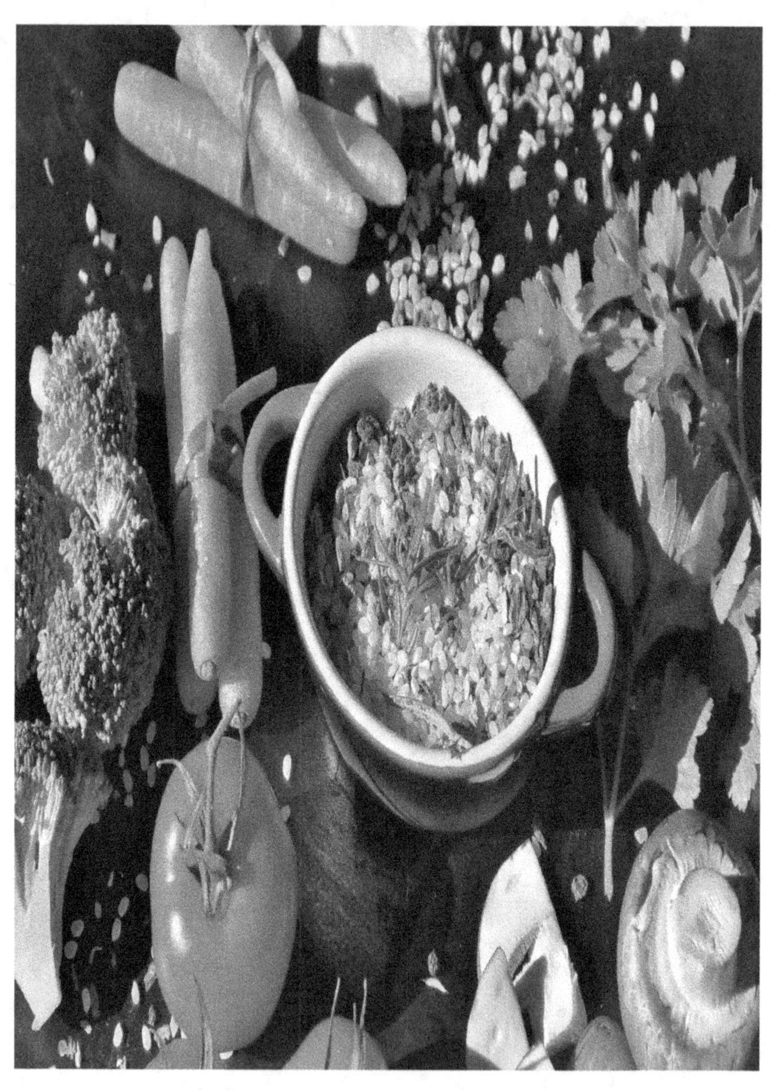

14.  Stuffed Bell Peppers with Lentils & Rice:

Ingredients:

- Bell peppers (any color)
- 1 cup cooked brown rice
- 1 cup cooked lentils
- 1/2 cup diced tomatoes
- 1/4 cup diced red onion
- 1/4 cup chopped fresh parsley
- 1 clove garlic, minced
- 1 teaspoon ground cumin
- Salt and pepper to taste

Preparation:

Preheat the oven to 375°F (190°C). Cut the tops off bell peppers and remove seeds and membranes.

In a large mixing bowl, combine cooked brown rice, cooked lentils, diced tomatoes, diced red onion, chopped parsley, minced garlic, ground cumin, salt, and pepper.

Stuff each bell pepper with the rice and lentil mixture, pressing down gently to pack it in.

Place stuffed bell peppers in a baking dish and cover with foil.

Bake in the preheated oven for 25-30 minutes, or until the peppers are tender.

Serve hot, optionally topped with a dollop of dairy-free yogurt or salsa.

15.  Buddha Bowl:

Ingredients:

- Cooked quinoa or rice
- Assorted roasted vegetables (such as sweet potatoes, cauliflower, Brussels sprouts)
- Sliced avocado
- Cooked chickpeas or black beans
- Fresh greens (such as spinach or kale)
- Tahini or hummus for drizzling

Preparation:

Arrange cooked quinoa or rice, roasted vegetables, sliced avocado, cooked chickpeas or black beans, and fresh greens in a bowl.

Drizzle with tahini or hummus for added flavor.

Serve the Buddha bowl warm or at room temperature.

16.  Chickpea Curry:

Ingredients:

- 1 can chickpeas, drained and rinsed
- Assorted vegetables (such as bell peppers, cauliflower, peas)
- 1 can coconut milk
- Curry powder
- Turmeric
- Cumin
- Garlic powder
- Onion powder
- Salt and pepper
- Cooked rice or quinoa for serving

Preparation:

In a large skillet or pot, combine chickpeas, assorted vegetables, and coconut milk.

Season with curry powder, turmeric, cumin, garlic powder, onion powder, salt, and pepper to taste.

Bring the mixture to a simmer over medium heat and cook for 15-20 minutes until vegetables are tender and flavors are well combined.

Serve the chickpea curry over cooked rice or quinoa.

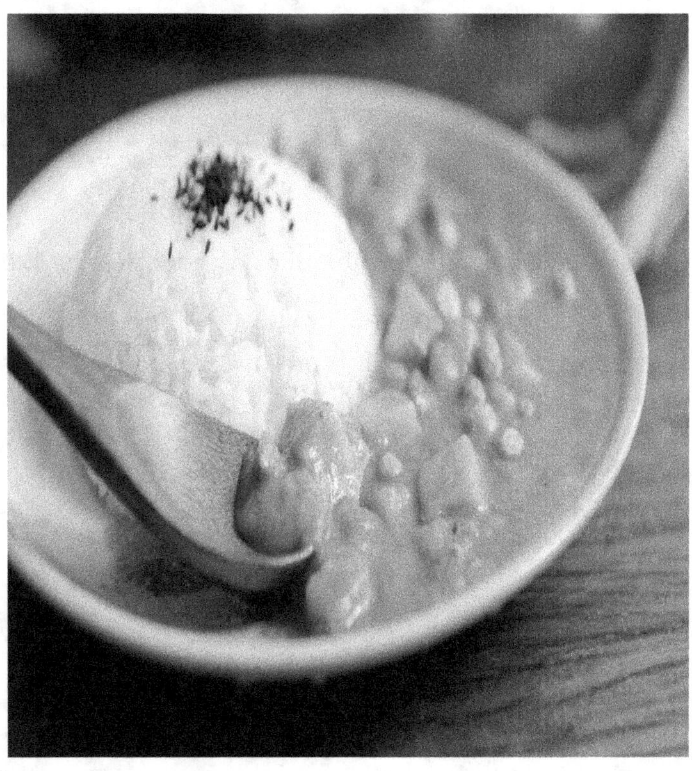

17. Spinach and Mushroom Quesadillas:

Ingredients:

- Gluten-free tortillas
- Fresh spinach leaves
- Sliced mushrooms
- Dairy-free cheese shreds
- Olive oil
- Salt and pepper

Preparation:

Heat a non-stick skillet over medium heat.

Brush one side of a gluten-free tortilla with olive oil and place it oil-side down in the skillet.

Layer dairy-free cheese shreds, fresh spinach leaves, and sliced mushrooms on one half of the tortilla.

To form a half-moon, fold the remaining tortilla over the filling.

Cook until crispy and golden brown, 2 to 3 minutes per side.

Repeat with remaining tortillas and filling ingredients.

Slice the quesadillas into wedges and serve hot.

18.  Falafel Bowl:

Ingredients:

- Baked or pan-fried falafel patties
- Cooked quinoa or rice
- Hummus
- Tzatziki sauce (vegan)
- Assorted chopped vegetables (such as cucumber, tomato, red onion)
- Fresh parsley or cilantro

Preparation:

Arrange cooked quinoa or rice in a bowl.

Top with baked or pan-fried falafel patties, hummus, and vegan tzatziki sauce.

Add assorted chopped vegetables on top.

Garnish with fresh parsley or cilantro.

Serve the falafel bowl warm or at room temperature.

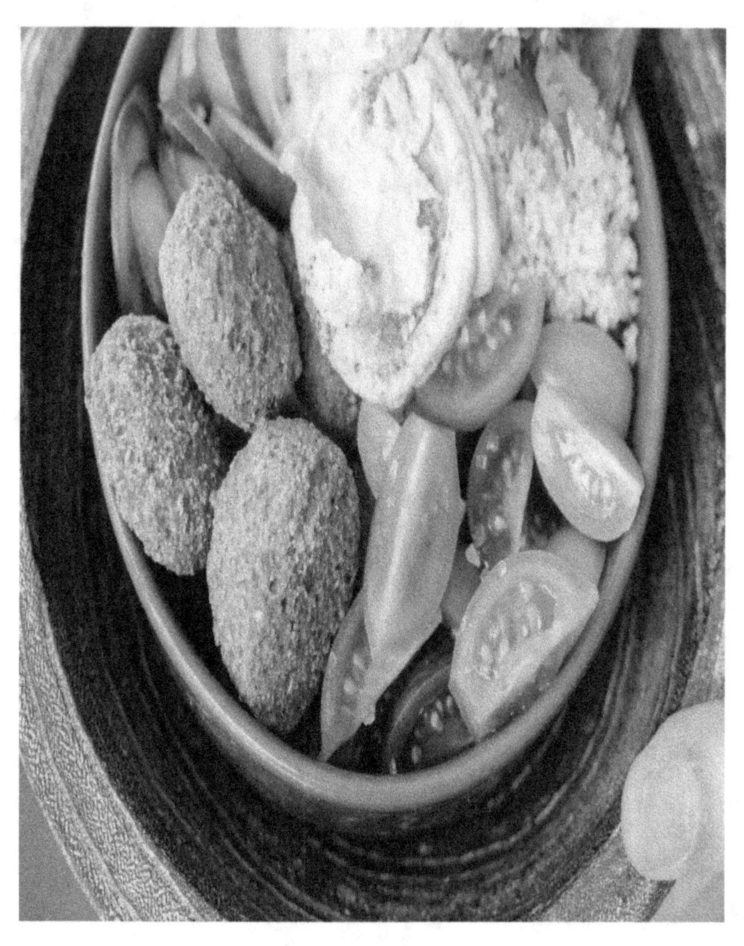

19.  cauliflower rice with salsa:

Ingredients:

For the cauliflower rice:

- 1 head of cauliflower
- 1 tablespoon olive oil
- Salt and pepper to taste

For the salsa:

- 2 large tomatoes, diced
- 1 small red onion, finely chopped
- 1 jalapeno pepper, seeded and finely chopped (adjust according to spice preference)
- 1/4 cup fresh cilantro, chopped
- Juice of 1 lime
- Salt and pepper to taste

Instructions:

Prepare the cauliflower rice by removing the leaves and core from the cauliflower head. Cut the cauliflower into florets.

In batches, pulse the cauliflower florets in a food processor until they resemble rice-like grains. Be careful not to over-process, as you don't want it to turn into a puree.

Heat olive oil in a large skillet over medium heat. Add the cauliflower rice to the skillet and sauté for 5-7 minutes, stirring frequently, until it's tender but not mushy. Season with salt and pepper to taste.

While the cauliflower rice is cooking, prepare the salsa. In a mixing bowl, combine the diced tomatoes, chopped red onion, jalapeno pepper, cilantro, lime juice, salt, and pepper. Mix well to combine.

Once the cauliflower rice is cooked, remove it from the heat and transfer it to a serving dish.

Serve the cauliflower rice topped with the freshly made salsa.

Enjoy your gluten-free vegan cauliflower rice with salsa as a tasty and nutritious meal or side dish!


20.  Avocado tomato salad:

Ingredients:

- 2 ripe avocados, diced
- 2 large tomatoes, diced
- 1/4 cup red onion, finely chopped
- 1/4 cup fresh cilantro, chopped
- Juice of 1 lime
- 1 tablespoon olive oil
- Salt and pepper to taste

Instructions:

Start by preparing the avocados. Cut them in half, remove the pits, and scoop out the flesh. Dice the avocado flesh into bite-sized pieces.

Dice the tomatoes and finely chop the red onion and cilantro.

In a mixing bowl, combine the diced avocado, tomatoes, red onion, and cilantro.

Drizzle one lime's juice over the salad's ingredients. Pour some olive oil over it.

To taste, add more salt and pepper to the salad. Mix everything together gently until well combined..

Let the salad sit for a few minutes to allow the flavors to meld together.

Taste and adjust seasoning if necessary.

Serve the gluten-free vegan avocado tomato salad as a refreshing side dish or a light meal.

This salad is not only delicious but also packed with healthy fats, vitamins, and minerals from the avocados and tomatoes. Enjoy!

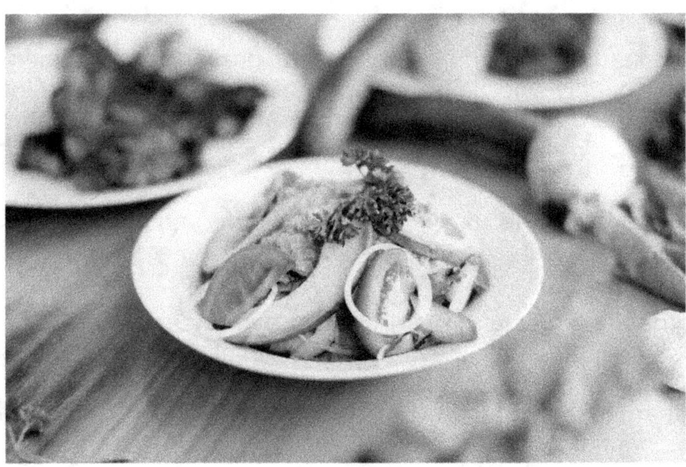

## 21.  Pear and Walnut Salad with Orange dressing:

Ingredients:

For the salad:

- 4 cups mixed salad greens (such as spinach, arugula, or mesclun)
- 2 ripe pears, thinly sliced
- 1/2 cup walnuts, toasted and chopped
- 1/4 cup dried cranberries or raisins

For the orange dressing:

- 1/4 cup freshly squeezed orange juice
- 2 tablespoons olive oil
- 1 tablespoon maple syrup or agave nectar
- 1 tablespoon Dijon mustard
- Salt and pepper to taste

Instructions:

Start by preparing the salad greens. Wash them thoroughly and spin them dry using a salad spinner or pat them dry with a clean kitchen towel. Place the salad greens in a large salad bowl.

Slice the pears thinly, removing the core and seeds. Add the sliced pears to the salad bowl with the greens.

Toast the walnuts in a dry skillet over medium heat for a few minutes until they become fragrant. Be careful not to burn them. Once toasted, chop the walnuts and add them to the salad bowl.

Add the dried cranberries or raisins to the salad bowl with the other ingredients.

In a small bowl, whisk together the orange juice, olive oil, maple syrup or agave nectar, Dijon mustard, salt, and pepper until well combined. This will be your dressing.

Drizzle the dressing over the salad in the salad bowl.

Gently toss the salad until all the ingredients are coated with the dressing.

Serve the gluten-free vegan pear and walnut salad immediately as a side dish or light meal.

This salad is bursting with flavor and textures, making it a perfect combination of sweet, savory, and crunchy. Enjoy!

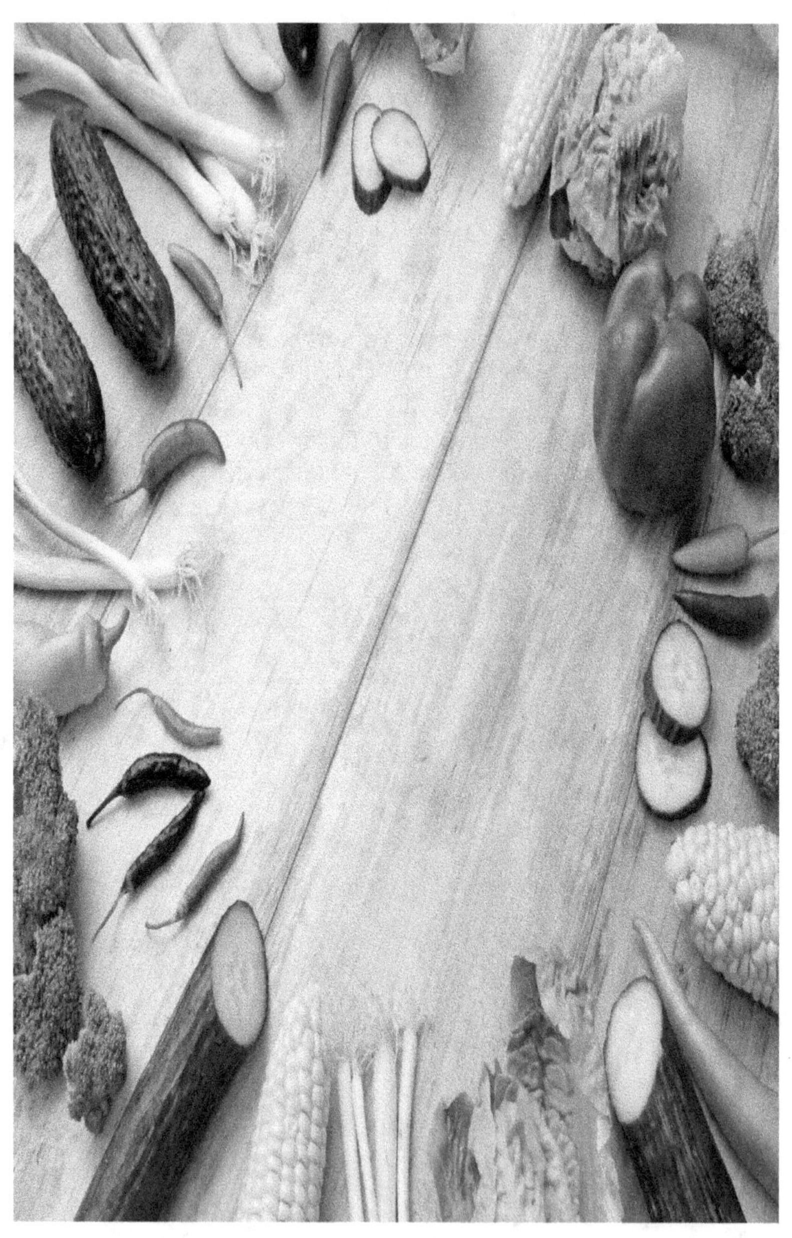

1. Lentil Bolognese

Ingredients:

- 1 cup dried green lentils, rinsed
- 2 tablespoons olive oil
- 1 onion, diced
- 2 cloves garlic, minced
- 1 carrot, diced
- 1 celery stalk, diced
- 1 can diced tomatoes
- 2 tablespoons tomato paste
- 1 teaspoon dried oregano
- 1 teaspoon dried basil
- Salt and pepper to taste
- Cooked gluten-free pasta of choice

Preparation:

Cook lentils according to package instructions and set aside.

In a large skillet, heat olive oil over medium heat. Add onion, garlic, carrot, and celery. Cook until softened.

Stir in cooked lentils, diced tomatoes, tomato paste, oregano, basil, salt, and pepper. Simmer for 10-15 minutes.

Serve over cooked gluten-free pasta.

## 2. Vegetable Stir-Fry with Tofu

Ingredients:

- 1 block firm tofu, pressed and cubed
- 2 tablespoons tamari or soy sauce
- 1 tablespoon sesame oil
- 1 tablespoon olive oil
- 2 cloves garlic, minced
- 1 tablespoon ginger, grated
- 2 cups of mixed vegetables (such as, broccoli, bell peppers and snap peas)
- Cooked rice or quinoa for serving
- Sesame seeds for garnish

Preparation:

In a bowl, marinate cubed tofu in tamari or soy sauce for 15 minutes.

Heat sesame oil and olive oil in a large skillet or wok over medium heat. Add garlic and ginger. Cook for 1 minute until fragrant.

Add marinated tofu to the skillet. Cook until golden brown on all sides.

Add mixed vegetables to the skillet. Stir-fry until vegetables are tender-crisp.

Serve over cooked rice or quinoa, garnished with sesame seeds.

## 3. Vegan Mushroom Risotto

Ingredients:

- 1 tablespoon olive oil
- 1 onion, diced
- 2 cloves garlic, minced
- 8 oz mushrooms, sliced
- 1 cup arborio rice
- 1/2 cup white wine (optional)
- 4 cups vegetable broth
- Salt and pepper to taste
- Fresh parsley for garnish

Preparation:

Heat olive oil in a large saucepan over medium heat. Add onion and garlic. Cook until softened.

Add sliced mushrooms to the saucepan. Cook until mushrooms release their juices.

Stir in arborio rice. Cook for 1 minute until lightly toasted.

If using, add white wine to the saucepan. Cook until wine is absorbed.

Gradually add vegetable broth to the saucepan, 1/2 cup at a time, stirring frequently until absorbed before adding more.

Continue cooking and stirring until rice is creamy and cooked to al dente.

Season with salt and pepper to taste.

Serve hot, garnished with fresh parsley.

4.   Black beans and Quinoa Stuffed Bell Peppers:

Ingredients:

- Bell peppers
- Quinoa
- Black beans
- Corn
- Diced tomatoes
- Onion
- Garlic
- Cumin, paprika, salt, and pepper

Preparation:

Cook quinoa according to package instructions.

Sauté onions and garlic until translucent.

Mix cooked quinoa, black beans, corn, diced tomatoes, onions, garlic, and spices.

Stuff the mixture into halved bell peppers.

Bake at 375°F (190°C) for 25-30 minutes.

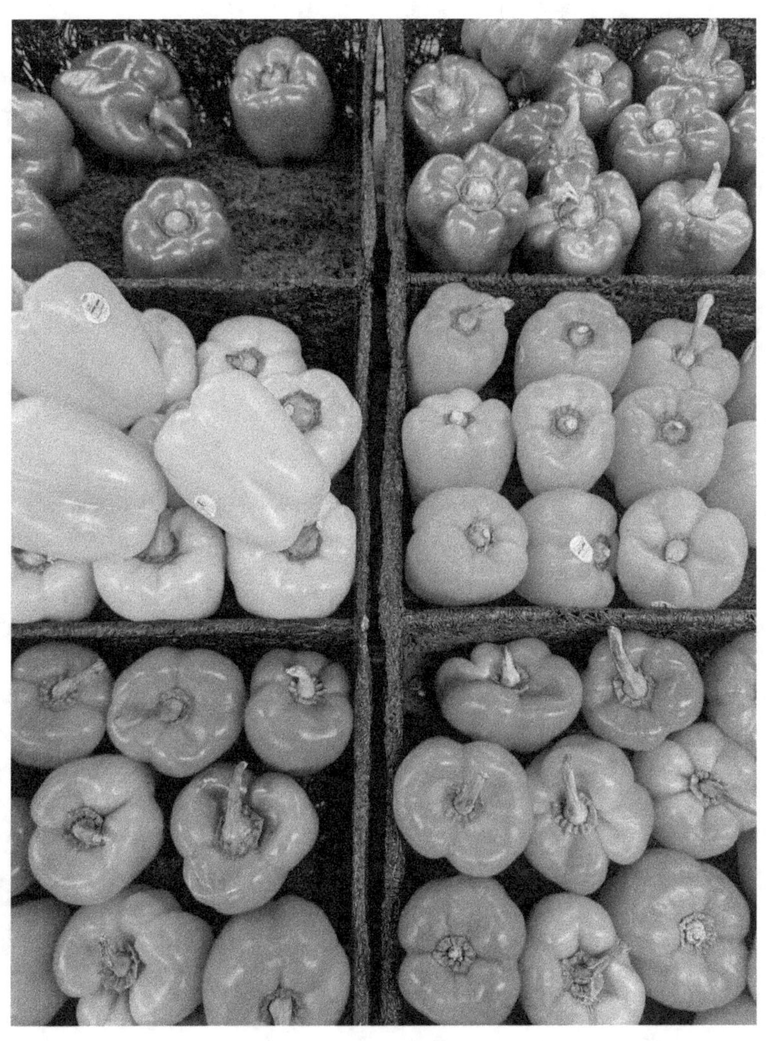

5.  Vegan Pad Thai:

Ingredients:

- Rice noodles
- Tofu
- Bell peppers
- Carrots
- Bean sprouts
- Green onions
- Garlic
- Lime
- Tamari or soy sauce
- Maple syrup

Preparation:

Cook rice noodles according to package instructions.

Sauté tofu, bell peppers, carrots, garlic, and green onions.

To the pan, add cooked noodles and bean sprouts.

Mix tamari or soy sauce with maple syrup and lime juice to make the sauce.

Pour the sauce over the noodles and vegetables and toss to combine thoroughly.

6. Chickpea and Vegetable Stir-Fry:

Ingredients:

- Chickpeas
- Broccoli
- Bell peppers
- Snow peas
- Carrots
- Onion
- Garlic
- Tamari or soy sauce
- Sesame oil

Preparation:

Sauté onions and garlic until fragrant.

Add chickpeas, broccoli, bell peppers, snow peas, and carrots.

Stir-fry until vegetables are tender.

Mix in tamari or soy sauce and a splash of sesame oil.

Serve over cooked rice or quinoa.

7.  Coconut Curry with Tofu:

Ingredients:

- Tofu
- Coconut milk
- Bell peppers
- Cauliflower
- Carrots
- Onion
- Garlic
- Curry powder
- Turmeric, salt, and pepper

Preparation:

Sauté onions and garlic until softened.

Add tofu, bell peppers, cauliflower, and carrots to the pan.

Stir in curry powder, turmeric, salt, and pepper.

Pour in coconut milk and simmer until vegetables are tender.

Serve over cooked rice or quinoa.

8. Mushroom and Spinach Risotto:

Ingredients:

- Arborio rice
- Mushrooms
- Spinach
- Vegetable broth
- Onion
- Garlic
- White wine (optional)
- Nutritional yeast (optional)

Preparation:

Sauté onions and garlic until translucent.

Add mushrooms and cook until browned.

Stir in arborio rice and cook for a few minutes.

Pour in white wine and cook until absorbed (if using).

Gradually add vegetable broth, stirring constantly, until rice is cooked.

Stir in spinach and nutritional yeast (if using) until wilted.

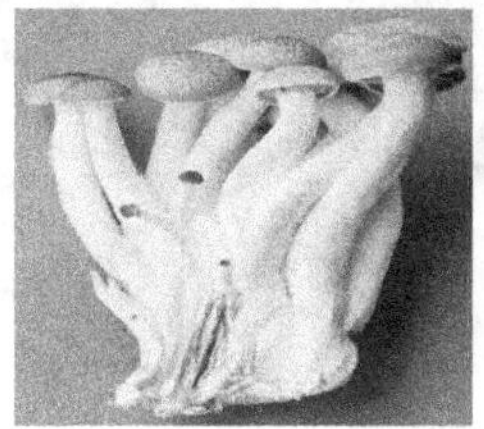

9. Vegan Chili:

Ingredients:

- Kidney beans
- Black beans
- Diced tomatoes
- Bell peppers
- Onion
- Garlic
- Chili powder
- Cumin, paprika, salt, and pepper

Preparation:

Sauté onions and garlic until softened.

Add bell peppers, diced tomatoes, kidney beans, and black beans.

Season with chili powder, cumin, paprika, salt, and pepper.

Simmer for 20-30 minutes.

Serve with avocado slices and chopped cilantro.

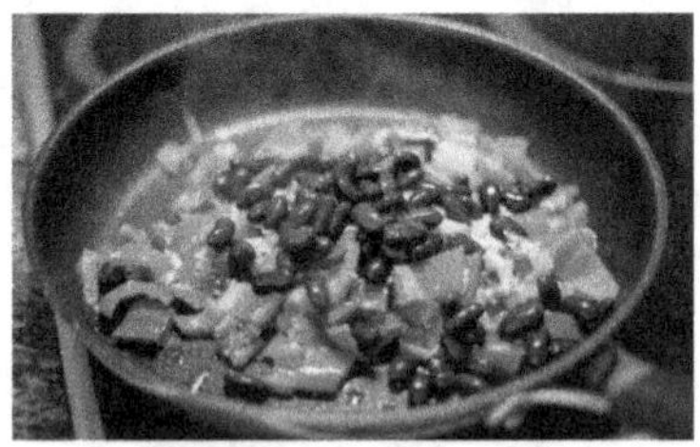

10. Vegan Buddha Bowl:

Ingredients:

- Quinoa
- Chickpeas
- Roasted sweet potatoes
- Steamed broccoli
- Sliced cucumber
- Avocado
- Tahini dressing (tahini, lemon juice, garlic, water)

Preparation:

Cook quinoa according to package instructions.

Roast sweet potatoes and chickpeas until crispy.

Steam broccoli until tender.

Arrange quinoa, sweet potatoes, chickpeas, broccoli, cucumber, and avocado in bowls.

Drizzle with tahini dressing before serving.

11. Vegan Mushroom Tacos:

Ingredients:

- Corn tortillas
- Mushrooms
- Red cabbage
- Avocado
- Cilantro
- Lime
- Garlic
- Cumin, paprika, salt, and pepper

Preparation:

Sauté mushrooms and garlic until browned.

Season with cumin, paprika, salt, and pepper.

Warm corn tortillas.

Fill tortillas with cooked mushrooms, sliced red cabbage, avocado, and cilantro.

Squeeze lime juice over the tacos before serving.

## 12. Vegan Ratatouille:

Ingredients:

- Eggplant
- Zucchini
- Bell peppers
- Onion
- Garlic
- Diced tomatoes
- Fresh basil
- Olive oil
- Salt and pepper

Preparation:

Sauté onions and garlic until softened.

Add diced tomatoes and simmer for a few minutes.

Layer sliced eggplant, zucchini, and bell peppers in a baking dish.

Pour the tomato mixture over the vegetables.

Drizzle with olive oil and season with pepper and salt.

Bake at 375°F (190°C) for 45-50 minutes, until vegetables are tender.

Garnish with fresh basil before serving.

13.  Cauliflower Curry:

Ingredients:

- Cauliflower
- Coconut milk
- Chickpeas
- Onion
- Garlic
- Ginger
- Curry powder
- Turmeric
- Cumin

Preparation:

Sauté onions, garlic, and ginger until softened.

Add cauliflower florets and chickpeas to the pan.

Stir in curry powder, turmeric, and cumin.

Pour in coconut milk and simmer until cauliflower is tender.

Serve over rice or quinoa.

14. Zucchini Noodles with Avocado Pesto:

Ingredients:

- Zucchini
- Avocado
- Basil
- Lemon juice
- Garlic
- Pine nuts
- Salt and pepper

Preparation:

Spiralize zucchini into noodles.

Blend avocado, basil, lemon juice, garlic, and pine nuts until smooth.

Toss zucchini noodles with avocado pesto.

Season with salt and pepper to taste.

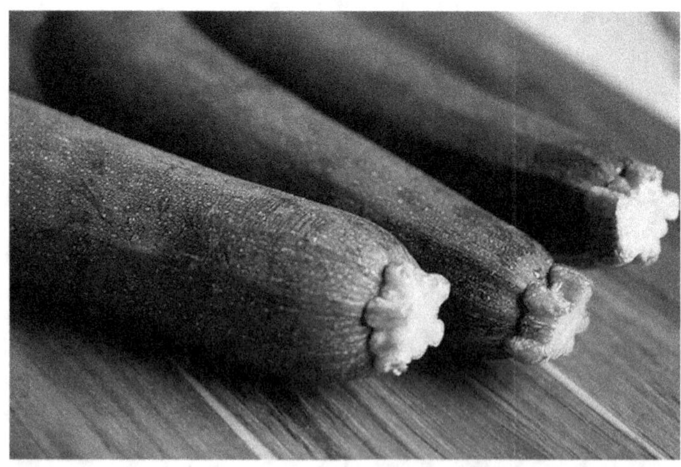

15.  Sweet Potato and Black Bean Enchiladas:

Ingredients:

- Sweet potatoes
- Black beans
- Corn tortillas
- Enchilada sauce (check for gluten-free)
- Onion
- Garlic
- Cumin
- Chili powder

Preparation:

Roast sweet potatoes until tender, then mash them with black beans, sautéed onions, garlic, cumin, and chili powder.

Fill corn tortillas with the sweet potato-black bean mixture.

Roll up tortillas and place them in a baking dish.

Pour enchilada sauce over the top.

Bake at 350°F (175°C) for 20-25 minutes.

16. Chickpea Salad with Lemon-Tahini Dressing:

Ingredients:

- Chickpeas
- Cucumber
- Cherry tomatoes
- Red onion
- Parsley
- Tahini
- Lemon juice
- Garlic
- Olive oil

Preparation:

Rinse and drain chickpeas, then toss them with chopped cucumber, cherry tomatoes, red onion, and parsley.

In a separate bowl, whisk together tahini, lemon juice, minced garlic, and olive oil to make the dressing.

Pour the dressing over the chickpea salad and toss to mix.

17. Stuffed Portobello Mushrooms:

Ingredients:

- Portobello mushrooms
- Quinoa
- Spinach
- Sun-dried tomatoes
- Pine nuts
- Garlic
- Balsamic vinegar

Preparation:

Remove stems from portobello mushrooms and clean them.

Cook quinoa according to package instructions.

Sauté spinach, sun-dried tomatoes, pine nuts, and minced garlic until spinach is wilted.

Mix cooked quinoa with the sautéed vegetables.

Stuff the portobello mushrooms with the quinoa mixture.

Drizzle with balsamic vinegar and bake at 375°F (190°C) for 15-20 minutes.

18. Vegetable Curry with Lentils:

Ingredients:

- Lentils
- Mixed vegetables (cauliflower, carrots, peas)
- Coconut milk
- Curry powder
- Onion
- Garlic
- Ginger

Preparation:

Cook lentils according to package instructions.

Sauté garlic, onions, and ginger until fragrant.

Add mixed vegetables to the pan and cook until slightly tender.

Stir in cooked lentils, curry powder, and coconut milk.

Simmer until vegetables are cooked through.


19.  Spaghetti Squash with Marinara Sauce:

Ingredients:

- Spaghetti squash
- Crushed tomatoes
- Onion
- Garlic
- Basil
- Oregano
- Olive oil

Preparation:

Preheat oven to 400°F (200°C). Cut spaghetti squash in half lengthwise and remove seeds.

Brush the inside with olive oil and place face down on a baking sheet.

Roast for 40-50 minutes, until squash is tender and can be easily shredded with a fork.

Sauté onions and garlic in olive oil until translucent.

Add crushed tomatoes, basil, oregano, salt, and pepper to the pan and simmer for 15-20 minutes.

Use a fork to shred the cooked spaghetti squash into strands.

Serve with marinara sauce on top.

20.  Vegan Lentil Shepherd's Pie:

Ingredients:

- Lentils
- Mixed vegetables (carrots, peas, corn)
- Onion
- Garlic
- Vegetable broth
- Potatoes
- Almond milk
- Vegan butter
- Thyme
- Rosemary

Preparation:

Cook lentils in vegetable broth until tender.

Sauté onions and garlic until softened, then add mixed vegetables and cook until tender.

Mix cooked lentils and vegetables together, season with thyme, rosemary, salt, and pepper.

Boil potatoes until soft, then mash with almond milk and vegan butter until smooth.

Spread the lentil and vegetable mixture into a baking dish, then spread the mashed potatoes on top.

Bake at 375°F (190°C) for 25-30 minutes, until the top is golden brown.

Enjoy these delicious gluten-free vegan dinner recipes!

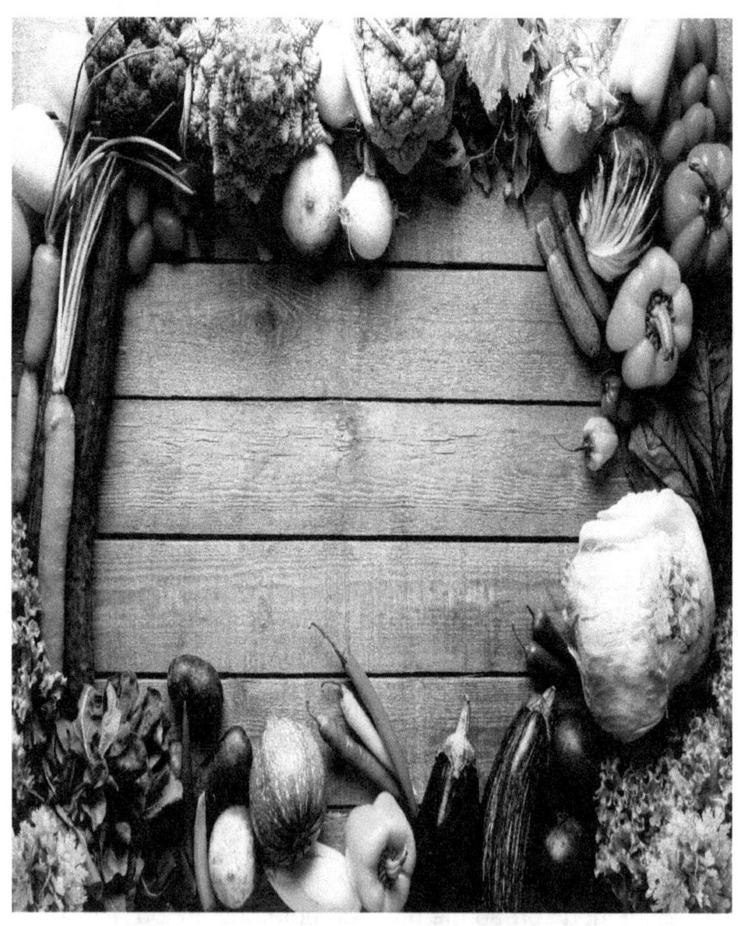

## 1. Chocolate Avocado Mousse

Ingredients:

- 2 ripe avocados
- 1/4 cup cocoa powder
- 1/4 cup maple syrup or agave nectar
- 1/4 cup almond milk (or any other plant-based milk)
- 1 teaspoon vanilla extract
- Optional toppings: chopped nuts, berries, coconut flakes

Preparation:

Cut the avocados in half, remove the pits, and scoop the flesh into a blender or food processor.

Add cocoa powder, maple syrup (or agave nectar), almond milk, and vanilla extract to the blender.

Blend the mixture until smooth and creamy, brushing down the sides as needed to ensure everything is well combined.

Taste the mousse and adjust sweetness if needed by adding more maple syrup or agave.

Transfer the mousse into serving bowls or glasses.

Put in the refrigerator to chill for at least 30 minutes before serving.

Garnish with your favorite toppings like chopped nuts, berries, or coconut flakes before serving.

2.  Coconut Mango Chia Pudding

Ingredients:

- 1/4 cup chia seeds
- 1 cup coconut milk
- 1 ripe mango, diced
- 1 tablespoon maple syrup or agave nectar (optional, depending on sweetness preference)
- Shredded coconut for garnish (optional)

Preparation:

Combine in a bowl, chia seeds and coconut milk. Stir well to combine.

Add maple syrup or agave nectar if desired for extra sweetness, and mix thoroughly.

Let the mixture sit for about 10 minutes, then stir again to prevent clumping.

Cover the bowl and refrigerate for at least 4 hours or overnight, allowing the chia seeds to absorb the liquid and thicken into a pudding-like consistency.

Once the chia pudding is set, spoon it into serving glasses or bowls.

Top the pudding with diced mango and shredded coconut.

Serve chilled and enjoy!

3.  Raw Vegan Brownies

Ingredients:

- 1 cup walnuts
- 1 cup dates, pitted
- 3 tablespoons cocoa powder
- Pinch of salt

Preparation:

Blend walnuts in a food processor, until finely ground.

Add dates, cocoa powder, and salt. Blend until the mixture sticks together.

Press the mixture into a lined baking dish and put in the refrigerator for at least an hour.

Cut into squares and serve.

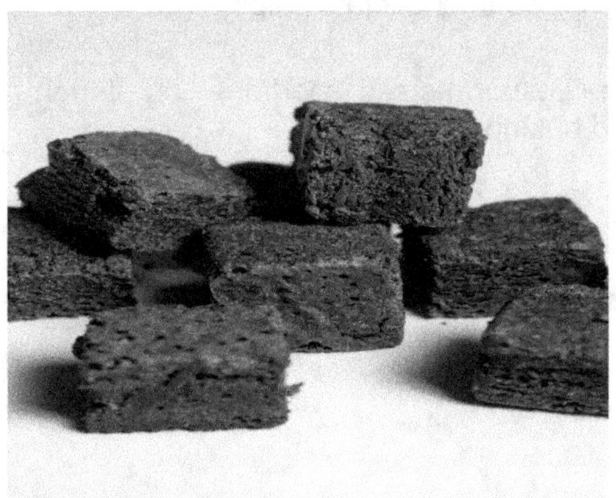

4. Vegan Chocolate Chip Cookies

Ingredients:

- 2 cups almond flour
- 1/4 cup maple syrup
- 1/4 cup coconut oil, melted
- 1 teaspoon vanilla extract
- 1/2 teaspoon baking soda
- 1/4 teaspoon salt
- 1/2 cup vegan chocolate chips

Preparation:

Preheat oven to 350°F (175°C) and line a baking sheet with parchment paper.

In a bowl, mix almond flour, maple syrup, melted coconut oil, vanilla extract, baking soda, and salt until well combined.

Fold in the vegan chocolate chips.

Place tablespoon-sized portions of dough on the prepared baking sheet.

Bake for 10–12 minutes, or until lightly golden.

Allow to cool on the baking sheet for 5 minutes before moving to a wire rack to cool completely..

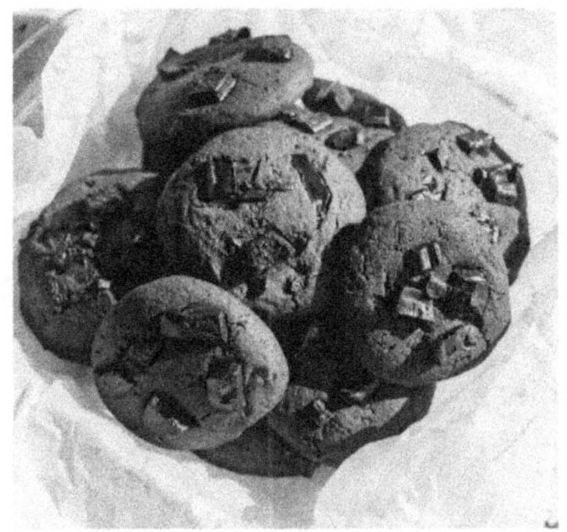

## 5. Coconut Date Balls

Ingredients:

- 1 cup Medjool dates, pitted
- 1 cup shredded coconut
- 1/2 cup almonds
- 1 tablespoon coconut oil
- 1/2 teaspoon vanilla extract

Preparation:

In a food processor, blend dates, shredded coconut, almonds, coconut oil, and vanilla extract until the mixture sticks together.

Roll the mixture into balls using your hands.

Roll the balls in additional shredded coconut if desired.

Refrigerate for at least 30 minutes before serving.

## 6.  Berry Quinoa Parfait

Ingredients:

- 1 cup cooked quinoa, cooled
- 1 cup mixed berries (such as strawberries, blueberries, raspberries)
- 1/2 cup coconut yogurt
- 2 tablespoons maple syrup or agave nectar
- 1/4 cup shredded coconut

Preparation:

In a bowl, mix cooked quinoa with maple syrup or agave nectar.

In serving glasses, layer quinoa, coconut yogurt, and mixed berries.

Repeat layers until glasses are filled.

Top with shredded coconut before serving.

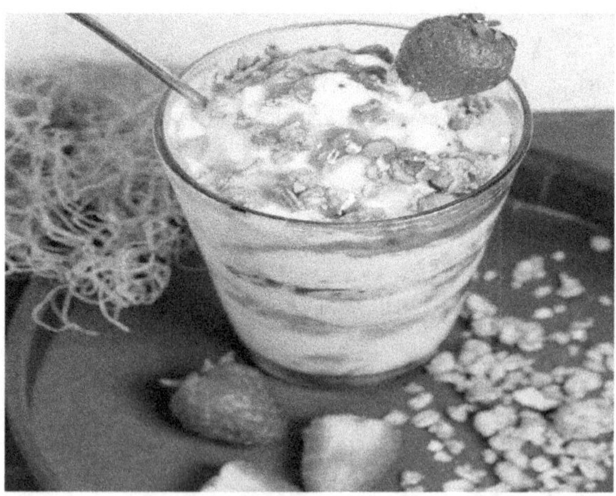

7.  Vegan Rice Crispy Treats

Ingredients:

- 4 cups gluten-free crispy rice cereal
- 1/2 cup brown rice syrup
- 1/2 cup almond butter
- 1 teaspoon vanilla extract

Preparation:

In a large mixing bowl, combine crispy rice cereal and almond butter.

In a small saucepan, heat brown rice syrup over medium heat until warm.

Stir in vanilla extract.

Pour the warm syrup mixture over the rice cereal and almond butter mixture.

Stir until cereal is evenly coated and well combined.

Press the mixture into a lined baking dish.

Let cool completely before cutting into squares.

## 8.  Chocolate Coconut Truffles

Ingredients:

- 1 cup shredded coconut
- 1/4 cup cocoa powder
- 1/4 cup maple syrup
- 2 tablespoons coconut oil, melted
- 1/2 teaspoon vanilla extract

Preparation:

In a bowl, mix shredded coconut, cocoa powder, maple syrup, melted coconut oil, and vanilla extract until well combined.

With your hands, roll the mixture into small balls.

If desired, roll the balls in more shredded coconut.

Let it cool for a minimum of half an hour before serving.

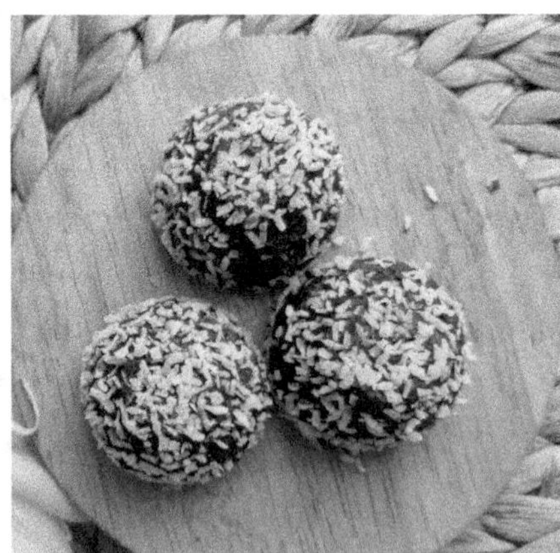

9. Peanut Butter Banana Ice Cream

Ingredients:

- 4 ripe bananas, sliced and frozen
- 2 tablespoons peanut butter
- 1 tablespoon maple syrup or agave nectar (optional)

Preparation:

In a blender or food processor, blend frozen banana slices, peanut butter, and maple syrup until smooth and creamy.

You can freeze it for a firmer texture or serve it immediately as soft-serve ice cream.

Optional: Top with chopped nuts or vegan chocolate chips before serving.

10. Vegan Apple Crisp

Ingredients:

- 4 apples, peeled, cored, and sliced
- 1 tablespoon lemon juice
- 1/4 cup maple syrup or agave nectar
- 1 teaspoon ground cinnamon
- 1 cup gluten-free rolled oats
- 1/2 cup almond flour
- 1/4 cup coconut oil, melted
- 1/4 cup chopped nuts (optional)

Preparation:

Preheat the oven to 350°F (175°C) and grease a baking dish.

In a bowl, toss apple slices with lemon juice, maple syrup, and cinnamon until well coated.

Transfer the apple mixture to the prepared baking dish.

In a separate bowl, combine rolled oats, almond flour, melted coconut oil, and chopped nuts (if using). Mix until crumbly.

Spread the oat mixture evenly over the apples in the baking dish.

Bake for 30-35 minutes or until the topping is golden brown and the apples are tender.

Let cool slightly before serving. Serve warm with a scoop of dairy-free ice cream or coconut whipped cream if desired.

11. Raw Vegan Lemon Bars

Ingredients:

For the crust:

- 1 cup raw almonds
- 1 cup dates, pitted

For the filling:

- 1 1/2 cups cashews, soaked for about 4-6 hours

- 1/2 cup coconut cream
- 1/3 cup lemon juice
- Zest of 1 lemon
- 1/4 cup maple syrup or agave nectar
- 1/4 cup melted coconut oil

Preparation:

In a food processor, blend almonds and dates until crumbly and sticky.

Press the mixture into the bottom of a lined baking dish to form the crust.

In a blender, combine soaked cashews, coconut cream, lemon juice, lemon zest, maple syrup, and melted coconut oil. Blend until smooth.

Pour the filling on the crust and spread evenly.

Put in the Refrigerator for at least 4 hours or until set.

Cut into bars and serve chilled.

## 12.  Vegan Chocolate Peanut Butter Cups

Ingredients:

- 1 cup dairy-free chocolate chips
- 1/4 cup peanut butter
- Sea salt (optional)

Preparation:

Use silicone or paper liners to line a mini muffin pan.

Melt the chocolate chips in 30-second increments in a microwave-safe bowl, stirring in between, until smooth.

Spoon a small amount of melted chocolate into each muffin cup, spreading it up the sides.

Place the muffin tin in the freezer for at least 10 minutes to set.

Remove from the freezer and add a dollop of peanut butter into each cup.

Top with remaining melted chocolate, covering the peanut butter.

Sprinkle with sea salt if desired.

Return to the freezer for another 20-30 minutes until set.

Once set, remove the cups from the muffin tin and store in an airtight container in the refrigerator.

## 13.  Chia Seed Chocolate Pudding

Ingredients:

- 1/4 cup chia seeds
- 1 cup coconut milk
- 2 tablespoons cocoa powder
- 2 tablespoons maple syrup or agave nectar

Preparation:

In a bowl, whisk together chia seeds, coconut milk, cocoa powder, and maple syrup until well combined.

Let the mixture sit for 5 minutes, then whisk again to prevent clumping.

Cover the bowl and refrigerate for at least 2 hours or overnight, allowing the chia seeds to absorb the liquid and thicken into a pudding-like consistency.

Serve chilled with toppings like fresh fruit or coconut flakes.

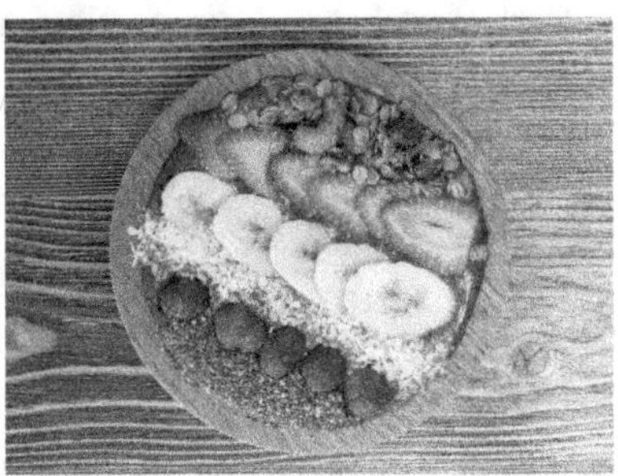

14. Vegan Banana Bread

Ingredients:

- 3 ripe bananas, mashed
- 1/4 cup coconut oil, melted
- 1/4 cup maple syrup
- 1 teaspoon vanilla extract
- 2 cups gluten-free all-purpose flour
- 1 teaspoon baking powder
- 1/2 teaspoon baking soda
- 1/2 teaspoon cinnamon
- Pinch of salt

Preparation:

Oil a loaf pan and preheat the oven to 350°F (175°C).

Melted coconut oil, maple syrup, vanilla extract, and mashed bananas should all be combined in a big bowl.

In a separate bowl, whisk together gluten-free flour, baking powder, baking soda, cinnamon, and salt.

Stirring until just combined, gradually add the dry ingredients to the wet ingredients.

After the loaf pan is ready, pour the batter into it.

When a toothpick inserted into the center comes out clean, bake for 50 to 60 minutes.

After 10 minutes of cooling in the pan, move the food to a wire rack to finish cooling.

## 15.  Vegan Coconut Macaroons

Ingredients:

- 3 cups shredded coconut
- 1/2 cup coconut cream
- 1/4 cup maple syrup or agave nectar
- 1 teaspoon vanilla extract
- Pinch of salt

Preparation:

Adjust the oven temperature to 325°F (160°C) and place parchment paper on a baking sheet.

In a large bowl, mix together shredded coconut, coconut cream, maple syrup, vanilla extract, and salt until well combined.

Using a spoon or cookie scoop, form the mixture into small mounds and place them on the prepared baking sheet.

Bake for 20-25 minutes or until the macaroons are golden brown on the edges.

After a few minutes of cooling on the baking sheet, move the baked goods to a wire rack to finish cooling.

16.  Vegan Blueberry Crisp

Ingredients:

- 4 cups fresh or frozen blueberries
- 1 tablespoon lemon juice
- 1/4 cup maple syrup or agave nectar
- 1 cup gluten-free rolled oats
- 1/2 cup almond flour
- 1/4 cup coconut oil, melted
- 1/4 cup chopped nuts (optional)

Preparation:

Preheat the oven to 350°F (175°C) and grease a baking dish.

In a bowl, toss blueberries with lemon juice and maple syrup until well coated.

Spoon the blueberry mixture into the baking dish that has been ready.

In a separate bowl, combine rolled oats, almond flour, melted coconut oil, and chopped nuts (if using). Mix until crumbly.

Evenly cover the blueberries in the baking dish with the oat mixture.

Bake for 30-35 minutes or until the topping is golden brown and the blueberries are bubbling.

Let cool slightly before serving. If preferred, top warm servings with coconut whipped cream or dairy-free ice cream.

## 17. Vegan Pumpkin Pie

Ingredients:

- 1 1/2 cups pumpkin puree
- 1/2 cup coconut milk
- 1/4 cup maple syrup or agave nectar
- 2 tablespoons cornstarch or arrowroot powder
- 1 teaspoon vanilla extract
- 1 teaspoon ground cinnamon
- 1/2 teaspoon ground ginger
- 1/4 teaspoon ground nutmeg
- 1/4 teaspoon ground cloves
- Pinch of salt
- 1 gluten-free pie crust (store-bought or homemade)

Preparation:

Preheat the oven to 350°F (175°C) and prepare a gluten-free pie crust in a pie dish.

In a blender, combine pumpkin puree, coconut milk, maple syrup, cornstarch or arrowroot powder, vanilla extract, spices, and salt. Blend until smooth.

Pour the pumpkin mixture into the prepared pie crust.

Bake for 50-60 minutes or until the filling is set and the crust is golden brown.

Let cool completely before slicing and serving. Serve with dairy-free whipped cream if desired.

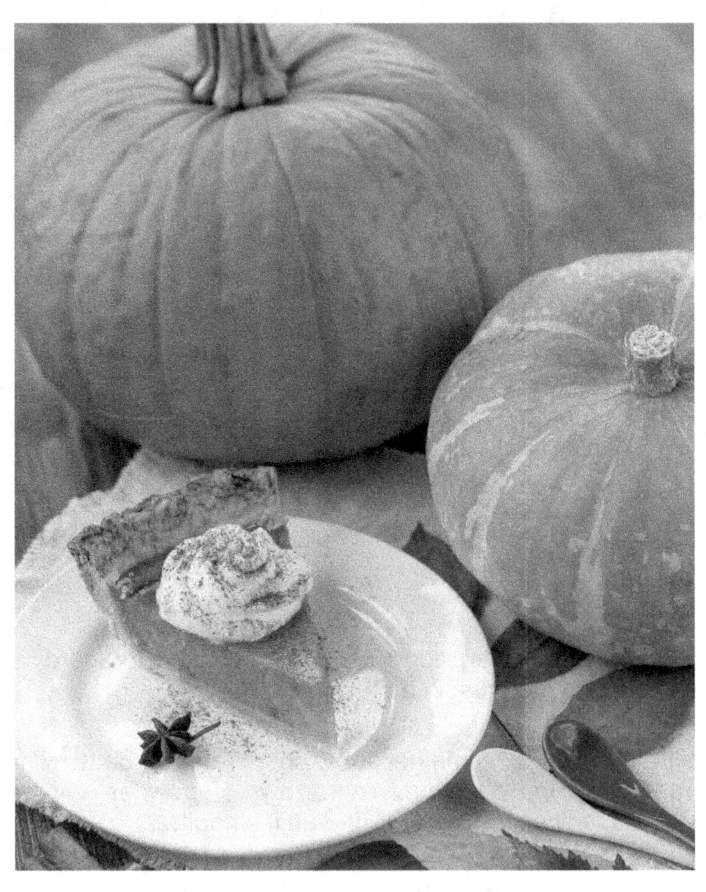

18. Vegan Raspberry Coconut Bars

Ingredients:

For the crust

- 1 cup gluten-free rolled oats
- 1 cup almonds
- 1/4 cup maple syrup
- 2 tablespoons coconut oil, melted
- Pinch of salt

For the Raspberry layer

- 2 cups fresh or frozen raspberries
- 2 tablespoons maple syrup
- 2 tablespoons chia seeds

For the Coconut toppings

- 1 cup shredded coconut
- 1/4 cup coconut milk
- 2 tablespoons maple syrup
- 1 tablespoon coconut oil, melted

Preparation:

Preheat oven to 350°F (175°C) and line a baking dish with parchment paper.

In a food processor, blend rolled oats and almonds until finely ground.

Add maple syrup, melted coconut oil, and a pinch of salt to the oat and almond mixture. Blend until well combined.

Press the mixture into the bottom of the lined baking dish to form the crust.

Bake for about 10-12 minutes or until lightly golden.

In a saucepan, combine raspberries and maple syrup. Cook over medium heat until mixture thickens slightly and the raspberries break down.

Remove from heat and stir in chia seeds. Let cool for a few minutes.

Pour the raspberry mixture over the baked crust and spread evenly.

In a bowl, mix together shredded coconut, coconut milk, maple syrup, and melted coconut oil to make the coconut topping.

Spread the coconut topping over the raspberry layer.

Bake for another 15-20 minutes or until the coconut topping is lightly golden.

Let cool completely before slicing into bars.

## 19.  Vegan Mango Sorbet

Ingredients:

- 3 cups frozen mango chunks
- 1/4 cup coconut milk
- 2 tablespoons maple syrup or agave nectar (optional, depending on sweetness of mango)
- 1 tablespoon lime juice (optional)

Preparation:

In a blender or food processor, blend frozen mango chunks, coconut milk, maple syrup or agave nectar, and lime juice until smooth.

If the mixture is too thick, you can add a little more coconut milk or water to help blend.

Once smooth, transfer the mixture to a shallow dish and freeze for at least 4 hours, stirring every hour to prevent ice crystals from forming.

Serve scoops of mango sorbet in bowls or cones.

## 20. Lemon Coconut Bliss Balls

Ingredients:
- 1 cup shredded coconut
- 1/4 cup coconut flour
- Zest and juice of 1 lemon
- 2 tbsp maple syrup

Preparation:
In a food processor, blend shredded coconut, coconut flour, lemon zest, lemon juice, and maple syrup until mixture sticks together.

Roll mixture into small balls and coat with extra shredded coconut if desired.

Refrigerate at least for 30 minutes before serving.


## 21. Pumpkin Spice Energy Bites

Ingredients:
- 1 cup rolled oats
- ½ cup pumpkin puree
- ¼ cup maple syrup
- 1 tbsp pumpkin pie spice
- ¼ cup chopped nuts (optional)

Preparation:

In a bowl, mix rolled oats, pumpkin puree, maple syrup, pumpkin pie spice, and chopped nuts until well combined.

Roll mixture into small balls and place on a baking sheet lined with parchment paper.

Chill in the refrigerator for 1 hour before serving.

## 22.  Chocolate Covered Strawberries

Ingredients:

- 1 pint fresh strawberries, washed and dried
- 1/2 cup dairy-free chocolate chips
- 1 tbsp coconut oil

Preparation:

Melt chocolate chips and coconut oil in 30-second increments in a microwave-safe bowl, stirring in between, until smooth.

Coat each strawberry halfway through by dipping it into the melted chocolate.

Place dipped strawberries on a parchment-lined baking sheet and refrigerate until chocolate is set

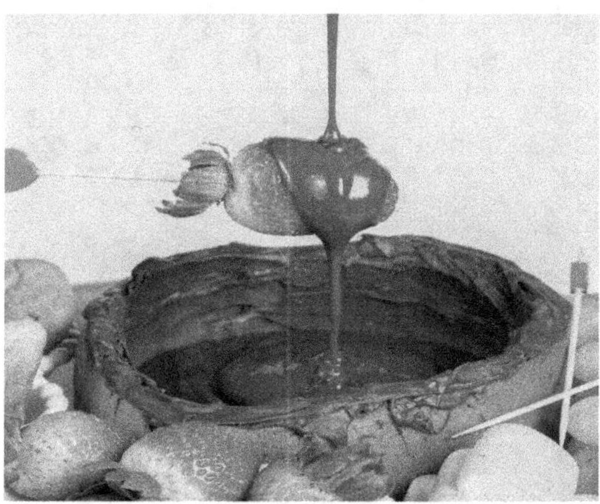

23. Chocolate Banana Oat Cookies

Ingredients:

- 2 ripe bananas, mashed
- 1 1/2 cups gluten-free rolled oats
- 1/4 cup cocoa powder
- 1/4 cup maple syrup
- 1/4 cup dairy-free chocolate chips

Preparation:

Preheat oven to 350°F (175°C) and line a baking sheet with parchment paper.

In a bowl, mix mashed bananas, rolled oats, cocoa powder, and maple syrup until well combined.

Fold in chocolate chips.

Drop spoonfuls of the mixture onto the prepared baking sheet and flatten slightly with a fork.

Bake for 12-15 minutes or until firm. Allow to cool before serving.

## 24.  Coconut Mango Popsicles

Ingredients:

- 2 ripe mangoes, peeled and diced
- 1 cup coconut milk
- 2 tbsp maple syrup
- 1/2 tsp vanilla extract

Preparation:

Blend diced mangoes, coconut milk, maple syrup, and vanilla extract until smooth.

Pour the mixture into popsicle molds.

Insert sticks and freeze for at least 4 hours or until firm.

Run molds under warm water to release popsicles before serving.


## 25.  Vegan Rice Krispie Treats

Ingredients:

- 4 cups gluten-free crispy rice cereal
- 1/2 cup brown rice syrup
- 1/2 cup almond butter
- 1/2 tsp vanilla extract

Preparation:

Grease a 9x9-inch baking dish and set aside.

In a large pot, heat brown rice syrup and almond butter over medium heat until melted and well combined.

Remove from heat, stir in vanilla extract, then add crispy rice cereal. Mix until evenly coated.

Fill baking dish with mixture, pressing firmly.

Allow to cool for one hour or more before slicing into squares.


## 26.  Strawberry Coconut Chia Pudding

Ingredients:

- 1/4 cup chia seeds
- 1 cup coconut milk
- 1 tbsp maple syrup
- 1/2 cup sliced strawberries

Preparation:

In a bowl, mix chia seeds, coconut milk, and maple syrup. Let sit for 10 minutes, then stir again.

Layer chia pudding and sliced strawberries in serving glasses.

Freeze for at least 2 hours or overnight before serving.

# 27. Apple Cinnamon Crumble

- Ingredients:
- 4 apples, peeled, cored, and sliced
- 1 tbsp lemon juice
- 1/2 cup almond flour
- 1/4 cup gluten-free rolled oats
- 1/4 cup coconut sugar
- 1 tsp cinnamon
- 2 tbsp coconut oil, melted

Preparation:
Preheat oven to 350°F (175°C) and grease a baking dish.

Toss sliced apples with lemon juice and spread evenly in the baking dish.

In a bowl, mix almond flour, rolled oats, coconut sugar, cinnamon, and melted coconut oil until crumbly.

Sprinkle the mixture over the apples.

Bake for about 35-40 minutes or until the topping is golden brown and the apples are tender.

Let cool slightly before serving.

These delightful gluten-free vegan dessert recipes offer a range of flavors and textures to satisfy any sweet tooth, all while adhering to dietary restrictions. Enjoy creating and indulging in these delicious treats!

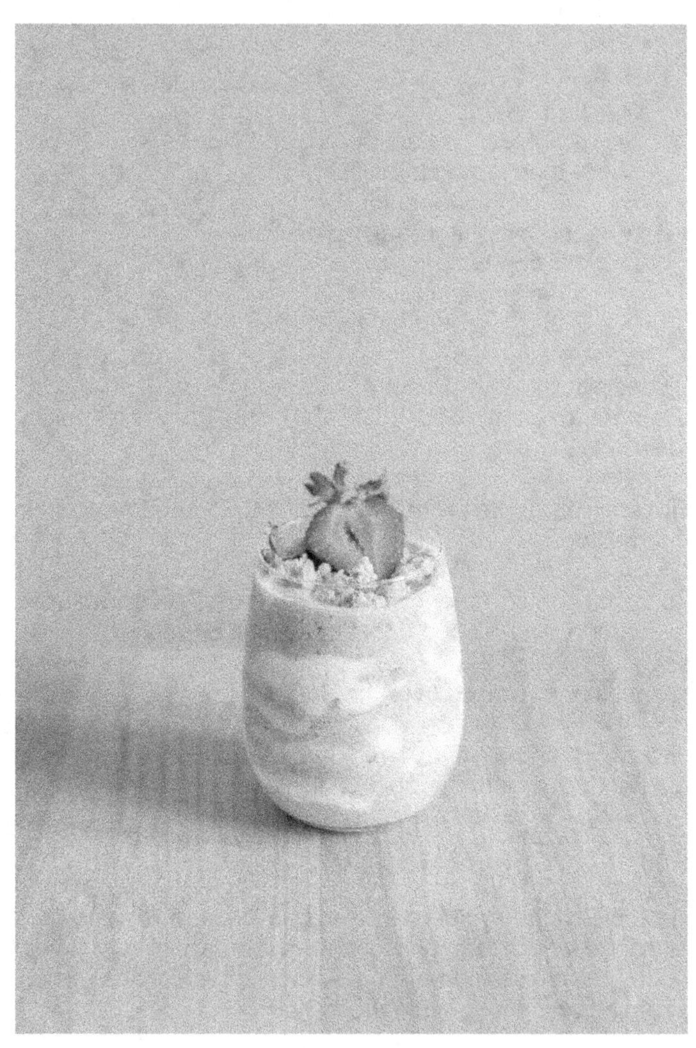

## 1. Chickpea Hummus

Ingredients:

- 1 can chickpeas, drained and rinsed
- 2 tablespoons tahini
- 2 tablespoons lemon juice
- 1 clove garlic, minced
- 2 tablespoons olive oil
- Salt and pepper to taste
- Optional toppings: paprika, chopped parsley, olive oil

Preparation:

In a food processor, combine chickpeas, tahini, lemon juice, garlic, and olive oil.

Blend until smooth, adding water as needed to achieve the desired consistency.

Season with salt and pepper to taste.

Transfer to a serving bowl, drizzle with olive oil, and sprinkle with paprika and chopped parsley if desired.

Serve with sliced vegetables, gluten-free crackers, or rice cakes.

2. Trail Mix

Ingredients:

- 1 cup mixed nuts (such as almonds, cashews, and walnuts)
- 1/2 cup dried fruit (like apricots, cranberries, and raisins)
- 1/4 cup seeds (such as pumpkin seeds and sunflower seeds)
- 1/4 cup dairy-free chocolate chips or carob chips (optional)

Preparation:

In a bowl, mix together mixed nuts, dried fruit, seeds, and chocolate chips.

Store in an airtight container or portion into individual snack bags for on-the-go snacking.

## 3. Roasted Chickpeas

Ingredients:

- 1 can chickpeas, drained and rinsed
- 1 tablespoon olive oil
- 1 teaspoon smoked paprika
- 1/2 teaspoon garlic powder
- 1/2 teaspoon onion powder
- Salt and pepper to taste

Preparation:

Preheat the oven to 400°F (200°C).

With a paper towel, pat dry the chickpeas to remove excess moisture.

In a bowl, toss chickpeas with olive oil, smoked paprika, garlic powder, onion powder, salt, and pepper.

Spread chickpeas in a single layer on a baking sheet lined with parchment paper.

Roast in the preheated oven for 20-25 minutes until crispy, shaking the pan halfway through baking.

Let cool before serving. Store in an airtight container.

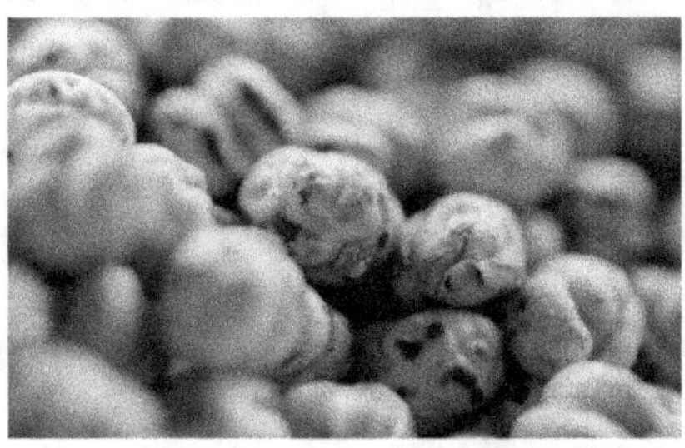

4.  Rice Cake with Almond Butter and Banana

Ingredients:

- Gluten-free rice cakes
- Almond butter (or any nut or seed butter)
- 1 ripe banana, sliced

Preparation:

Spread almond butter on top of a rice cake.

Top with sliced banana.

Enjoy as a quick and easy gluten-free vegan snack.


5.  Vegetable Sushi Rolls

Ingredients:

- Nori sheets
- Cooked sushi rice (made with rice vinegar, sugar, and salt)
- Assorted vegetables (such as cucumber, avocado, carrot, bell pepper)
- Tamari or soy sauce for dipping
- Pickled ginger and wasabi (optional)

Preparation:

Lay a sheet of nori on a sushi mat made of bamboo.

Over the nori sheet, evenly distribute the sushi rice, leaving a thin layer around the edges.

Arrange thinly sliced vegetables in a row across the rice.

Carefully roll up the nori sheet using the bamboo mat, pressing gently to seal.

Cut the sushi roll into bite-sized pieces using a sharp knife.

Serve with tamari or soy sauce for dipping, and pickled ginger and wasabi if desired.

6.  Quinoa Energy Balls:

Ingredients:

- 1 cup cooked quinoa
- 1/2 cup almond butter
- 1/4 cup maple syrup
- 1/4 cup shredded coconut
- 1/4 cup vegan chocolate chips

Preparation:

Mix all ingredients in a bowl until well combined.

Roll the mixture into balls.

Put in the fridge to set for at least 30 minutes.

7.  Roasted Spiced Nuts:

Ingredients:

- 2 cups mixed nuts (such as almonds, cashews, and walnuts)
- 1 tablespoon olive oil
- 1 teaspoon ground cumin
- 1 teaspoon smoked paprika
- 1/2 teaspoon garlic powder
- Salt to taste

Preparation:

Preheat oven to 350°F (175°C).

In a bowl, toss nuts with olive oil and spices until evenly coated.

Arrange the nuts in a single layer on a baking sheet.

Roast in the preheated oven for 10-15 minutes, or until fragrant and lightly browned.

8.  Crispy Kale Chips:

Ingredients:

- 1 bunch kale, washed and dried
- 1 tablespoon olive oil
- Salt to taste

Preparation:

Preheat oven to 275°F (135°C).

Tear kale leaves into bite-sized pieces, removing tough stems.

In a bowl, toss kale with olive oil and salt until evenly coated.

Spread kale in a single layer on a baking sheet.

Bake for 20-25 minutes, or until crispy.

9.   Raw Veggie Sticks with Hummus:

Ingredients:

- Carrot sticks
- Celery sticks
- Cucumber sticks
- Cherry tomatoes
- Hummus

Preparation:

Wash and cut vegetables into sticks.

Serve with hummus for dipping.

10.  Frozen Banana Bites

Ingredients:

- Ripe bananas, sliced
- Dairy-free chocolate chips
- Nut butter (optional)

Preparation:

Spread nut butter (if using) on banana slices.

Sandwich two banana slices together.

Dip each banana sandwich in melted dairy-free chocolate.

Place on a parchment-lined baking sheet and freeze until firm.

11.  Edamame Snack Pods

Ingredients:

- Edamame pods, steamed
- Sea salt

Preparation:

Steam edamame pods until tender.

Sprinkle with sea salt before serving.

These gluten-free vegan snack recipes are perfect for satisfying your cravings between meals or for an on-the-go energy boost! Enjoy making and snacking on them.

These recipes provide a variety of gluten-free vegan lunch options, from salads and sandwiches to hearty bowls and wraps. Enjoy experimenting with different flavors and ingredients to create satisfying and nutritious meals!

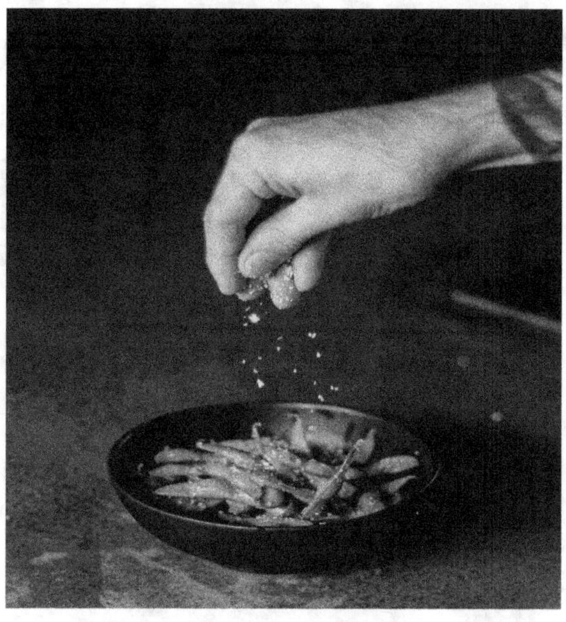

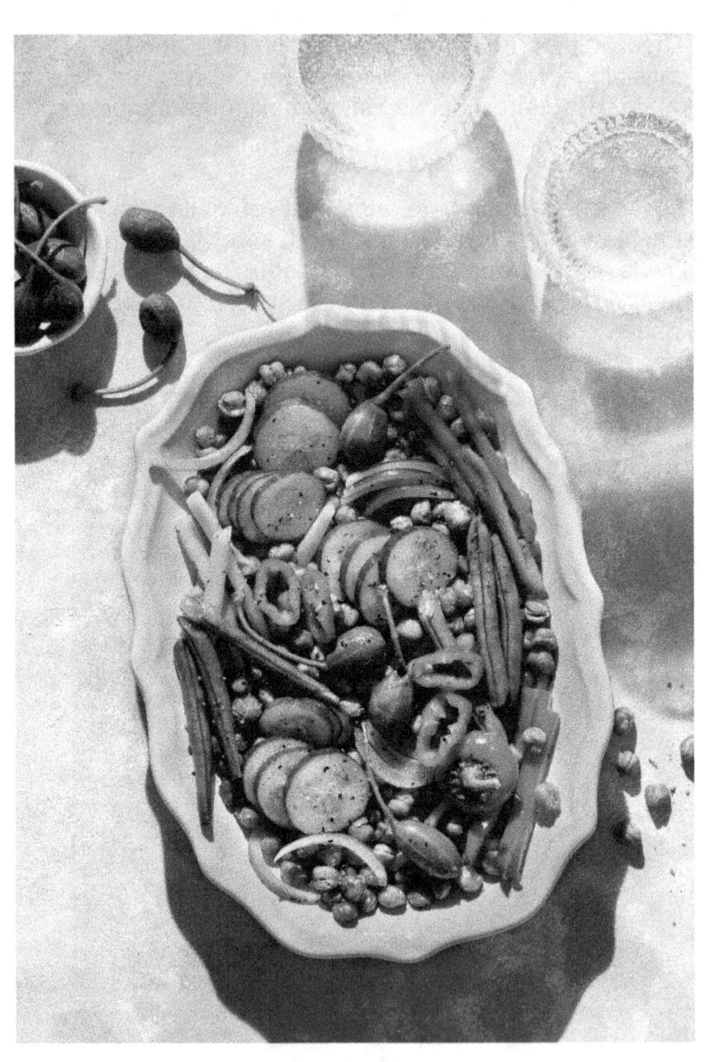

# CONCLUSION

In conclusion, the exploration of the gluten-free vegan lifestyle presented in this book illuminates not only the practicalities of dietary choices but also the profound impact such decisions can have on our health, the environment, and animal welfare. Through a comprehensive examination of recipes, nutritional insights, and personal anecdotes, it becomes evident that embracing a gluten-free vegan lifestyle is not merely a dietary adjustment but a transformative journey towards holistic well-being.

The book underscores the versatility and abundance of plant-based ingredients, demonstrating that eliminating gluten and animal products from one's diet need not equate to sacrificing flavor or variety. Instead, it opens up a world of culinary creativity and nourishment, offering an array of delicious and nutritious alternatives.

Moreover, beyond the kitchen, this lifestyle fosters a deeper connection with our food, encouraging mindfulness and intentionality in our consumption habits. By opting for plant-based, gluten-free options, we align ourselves with principles of sustainability and ethical stewardship, contributing to the preservation of our planet and the welfare of sentient beings.

Ultimately, the gluten-free vegan lifestyle advocated in this book empowers individuals to make informed choices that prioritize both personal wellness and broader environmental and ethical considerations. It serves as a roadmap for cultivating a more compassionate, healthful, and sustainable way of living, inspiring readers to embark on their own journey towards greater vitality, mindfulness, and harmony with the world around them.

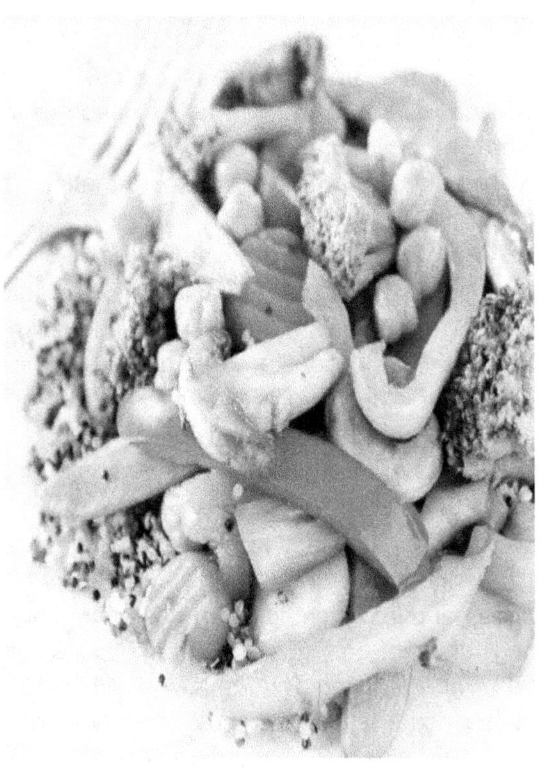